THE DIET

Nutrition is 90% of it; exercise is the other 50%.

Written by
Mike Horn and Rick Hoadley

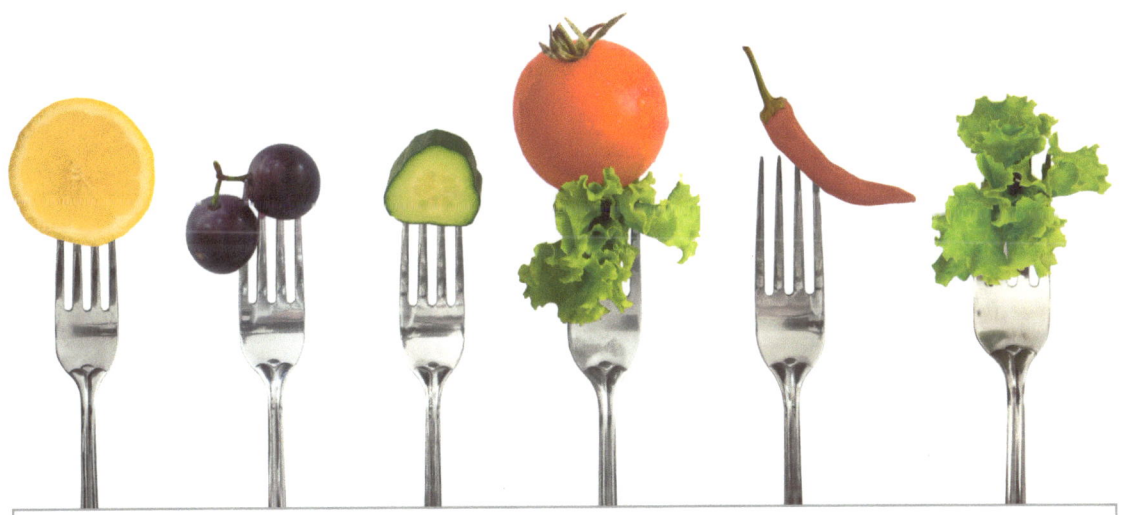

FOREWORD

The language in this book is not about losing, it's about gaining.

This book is straight talk-plain-simple-and direct. Explaining how to begin a plan, step-by-step, that will teach you how to control your body fat percentage.

This method can change your life in a positive manner, and can dramatically improve your health and quality of life, perhaps even your longevity.

Increased energy, a trimmer more attractive appearance and the boost in self-esteem, can help develop increased mental clarity and physical strength. These are all direct benefits of this life-style plan.

You can eliminate excess body fat, and gain understanding of how your muscles, nervous system, your metabolism and your spiritual self can be nourished and cared for.

We wish you much success in your new endeavors.

Mike Horn and Rick Hoadley

TABLE OF CONTENTS

Acknowledgements

Thank you to Master Tom Wasylyk for all your hard work, for seeing the big picture, and your attention to detail. Without you and your faith in the value of this project, it would not have come to pass.

Thank you to Mrs. Jan Horn, your support for Mike and myself has been essential, your expertise as a National Competitor in women's fitness and physique competition, as well as an expert personal trainer and business owner, has been extraordinary.

Thank you to Steve O'Brien, my dear friend, for all your input and editing.

Thank you to Karen Lepik, for all you have done, the infinite and unending list of things that must be done to keep everything together in the business and this project has been impossible, yet you have done it extremely well, God bless you for all you do.

Dreamstime.com - Photos on cover, title page, and pages 2, 4, 33, 34, 41, 44, 50, 51, and 52.

Bibliography

Sugar Blues by William Dufty Warner Books Edition is published by arrangement with Chilton Book Company, Chilton Way, Padnor, PA.,17089

Enter the Zone, Mastering The Zone by Barry Sears Ph.D., Harper Collins Publishers Inc., 10 East 53rd Street, New York , N.Y.

Protein Power by Michael R. Eades, M.D. and Mary Dan Eades, M.D. ISBN 0 - 553-57475-2 Library Of Congress catalogue card number 98-32738. Bantom Books a division of Bantom Doubleday Dell Publishing Group, Inc. Marca Registrada, Bantom Books1540 Broadway, New York, N.Y. 10036

How to Regulate Your Fat Thermostat - Authors: Parent, Remington, and Fischer

The Secret of Plants - Peter Thompson and Christopher Byrd, ISBN 0-06-014326-6 Harper and Row Publishers, New York, San Francisco, Evanston-London

Autobiography of a Yogi - Paranrahnasa Yoganando, Copyright©1982 Self-Realization Fellowship, Printed 1985

Power Sleep - Dr. James B. Maas

Nutrition is 90% of it. Exercise is the other 50%!

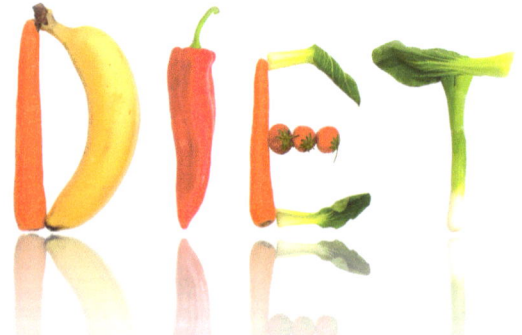

CHAPTER 1

THE LAST DIET BOOK
YOU WILL EVER NEED

You are tired of being fat! You have tried to lose weight but after a few days or weeks given up, and you felt even more discouraged than before, right?

This book is the answer. Deep inside don't you want to be that slim, trim, attractive, lean, sexy person you so richly deserve to be? How do these other people do it? And what is their secret?

Finally, here are the answers to these questions; how to do it: lose weight and make it work. How to maintain your weight where you want for the rest of your life, without the discouraging and often futile failure that you have experienced before! This is a book written because the information given here; as simple as it is, is not understood by the majority of the population. In this society of rampant and epidemic obesity, many people are offended or 'turned-off' by the suggestion that they stop eating certain foods. It's almost like they feel 'entitled' to eat whatever they want. This book will work if you follow directions EXACTLY.

The good news is that the changes you will make in your diet and lifestyle are small steps, but the synergy of coordinating these steps simultaneously will DRAMATICALLY change your metabolism, energy, and appearance. The information that will be revealed by this book can change your life, and the results will amaze you. This is definitely the last diet book you will ever need, and the real, practical knowledge you will learn will forever change your health and appearance, and you will enjoy the transformation that will improve your life in ways that will please and amaze you!

Many so-called professionals will take issue with much of what is presented to you in this book, making claims that this method is NOT scientific, even dangerous and unsafe, and not part of the accepted establishment theory of nutrition, diet, and exercise. Remember, books have been written that argue that the only way to lose weight and be healthy is to be a vegetarian, and books have been written that insist that you must eat ONLY meat, and no carbohydrate! These are diametrically opposed viewpoints, 180 degrees apart and in total disagreement and each theory containing some obvious elements of truth. A diet book has been written about foods that make you happy, and many books offer ridiculous and false claims that you can eat whatever you want. If only there was a magic pill? The truth is you need accurate information, and a plan proven to work by thousands of people.

This book is about balance, and doing what works!

The only people that will applaud this book are those who have followed the steps in this book, and the success enjoyed by those open-minded and intelligent people speaks for itself, and is its own reward.

I was eating at an 'All-You –Can –Eat' buffet restaurant one day and I sat next to a middle –aged white married couple who were eating their Sunday meal. They were both 50-75 # over-weight, and I made several observations as I ate my meal. I assumed that they were not well educated, and judging by their dress and appearance I also assumed that they were blue-collar workers. I made this determination based on their appearance, table manners, and pieces of their conversation that I heard. I assumed that the eating habits of these two people were learned from generation after generation of parents, grandparents, great grand parents, aunts and uncles, and other family members that ate food in a similar manner. Judging from the man's hands, he was a hard worker, probably getting up early every day and working long hours, and I assumed that his wife was either a homemaker or also employed. These two ate three plates that I observed, maybe more before and after I left the restaurant, and each plate was loaded with potatoes, mac-aroni, fried chicken, fried fish, steak, all covered with butter and cheese. Many rolls of bread were consumed, and all washed down with sweet tea. Hungry as I was that day, [I have the table manners of a timber wolf when I am famished!], these two ate with greater gusto than my-self and wolfed down plate after plate of starchy and sugary processed carbohydrates and fatty foods. The man ate so rapidly that when a macaroni noodle fell of his speeding fork, he did not miss a beat and scooped the noodle up with his fork, right off the shirt stretched over his ample and distended belly.

Now please understand me. I am not describing this scene to mock these two, or in any way be disrespectful. My heart is filled with compassion for these two and any people that suffer with obesity. These two are creatures in Christ, human beings deserving of dignity and respect. I assumed that they worked hard, paid taxes, probably raised a family, and were celebrating their after- church Sunday dinner in a low-priced restaurant that is noted for it's low price and endless supply of fattening, tasty, food. It is people like these two who are as Christ said in Matthew 5:13, "Ye are the salt of the Earth;"-these are the people who work the fields, toil with back-breaking labor, perform the many daily tasks necessary for our society to function, pay the taxes and purchases goods, products and services that drive our economy and upon which every business depends. Don't these people deserve a life of health? That bill of health includes a functioning, pain-free body that is endowed with the practical efficiency that God intended, a beautiful masterpiece created by God, in His image, and part of that grand and divine design. This body should not be dragging around an extra 20 or 30 pounds of unhealthy, unwanted fat, but these two, like millions in this country and around the world, don't know how to STOP the process of getting fat, and have no clue how to reverse this process and actually lose weight.

As I looked around the restaurant, I noticed that of the hundred or so people dining or wait-ing in line to eat, that dozens of these folks were obese. Corpulent, apple-shaped human beings weighing well over 200#, waddling around with huge thighs and behinds, and rolls of fat hanging over their belts, pendulant growths of fat rippling under their arms, double and triple chins, faces like basketballs, their expressions sad and empty, filled with emotional flatness and quiet desperation, attacking their food as a beaver gnaws at a tree trunk, chewing and chewing with a slow, methodical resignation that allows the consumer to eke out some nutritional sustenance and miserable pleasure that in a cruel , ironic joke torments and traps the poor unfortunate who endlessly repeats this vicious cycle of eating, getting fatter, becoming bigger and more ponderous, becoming hungry, eating, getting fatter, ad infinitum ad nauseaum. The man has got to eat, doesn't he? The trap is that the human lifestyle [and diet] in this country has changed in subtle yet profound ways. This eating is serious business, almost like feeding cattle, or alligators or sharks, and don't get in their way! In one hundred years we have evolved from consuming 4# of sugar per year to eating 170#, per year, from an agrarian nation where each family had a mule and 40 acres, their own milk cow, a small chicken coop, and a Victory garden, survived the Great Crash and Depression, and kicked global butt in WWII to a nation of morbidly obese, lazy, non-productive, poorly educated factory workers who got whipped in Viet Nam, are raising kids addicted to video games and drugs, can't compete with the Japanese auto makers, and are suckers for Arabian oil and afraid to go to war with Islamic terrorists who flatly declare that they intend to kill us all! As a country, we can't figure out this eating/ fat thing. This book is a plea to each every reader to search your own soul, and decide, is it important that you LEARN how to eat and exercise? So that you don't look like Jabba the Hut, and you don't feel like a hopeless, sloppy   Roman citizen too fat and weak to fight the Mongol and Vandal invaders that sacked and burned Rome.

This diet/ eating plan/ lifestyle- transfusion will change you in 90 days in ways that cannot be explained by current science or publications. You will kick-start your metabolism, come face-to face with your own comfort- zone/addiction slave-to flavor issues, and actually lose more body fat safely and quicker than any other diet or eating plan available today. If you are morbidly obese, or too fat, or just tired of being a 20# overweight Pillsbury Doughboy version of the trim, lean, svelte person you have secretly longed to be, read on, and make the decision to do this diet, because it works, and will move you physically, metabolically, and psychologically closer to the person you deserve to be. The only way this diet will fail you is if you don't begin, or quit before 90 days. At 90 days you will have learned first-hand, empirically, what works for you, and no matter how much you love food, you will have safely gained a perspective and distance from old habits, and a clarity that will change your awareness and decision making regarding the cause-and effect of food and eating. Almost like an alcoholic or drug addict gains distance and perspective and clarity concerning substance abuse after they have completed a 90 day rehabilitation program, you will gain valuable and practical knowledge about how you eat, and gain or lose body fat and muscle. I promise you will be glad you made this decision.

The language used in this book is very real, and the language may offend you. Mike and I both agree, we do not wish to offend anyone. Obesity is a serious problem, and many experts think that 66% of the adult population in this country is obese. The language, and the math, in this book are real simple, and plain. Obesity KILLS people, and makes people MISERABLE, and we ALL PAY for the medical costs involved, either by taxes, higher insurance premiums, and a clogged, overcrowded medical care system. If you were one of Mike's clients, or one of my Taekwondo or Jujutsu students, you would hear identical language. Any good coach will speak with passion and emotion, and taken out of context, someone listening may be offended by the plain talk, tone of voice, and choice of words. If you were an alcoholic, or drug addict, and you were involved in a quality rehabilitation program, you might hear some harsh language directed toward your behavior. "Love the sinner, HATE the sin!" is the operative thought in these situations. A drill Instructor training soldiers the tactics, techniques, and strategy of a dangerous military mission might use strong language, also. All of these situations are a matter of life-or -death, and if losing 10 or more pounds of unwanted fat is not a matter of life-or-death for you, then continue living the lifestyle that makes you fat, and your obesity will snowball gradually and afflict you with all the attendant diseases that are discussed in association with obesity. For a serious bodybuilder or Taekwondo or Jujutsu Instructor, FAILURE IS NOT AN OPTION! Same for a soldier engaged in a combat mission. Many alcoholics refer to themselves during therapy and counseling sessions as 'drunks'. Taken out of context, this term can be viewed as derogatory. However, during the actual session, the use of this term elicits an honest and objective glimpse of how other people who witness the destructive behavior of an active alcoholic see; and what the reality and consequences of such behavior are. The general population looks at an overweight person and thinks, "fat slob." A competent Drill Instructor in the Military also has witnessed the lethal consequence of a soldier's failure to complete the assignment, REGARDLESS of the excuse. In these situations, people die. With obesity, people also die, but first they suffer, horribly and needlessly, for years, before they succumb to a horrible combination of diseases. So, if you are man enough, or woman enough, or human enough, to read this book, there is hope for you.

The assault on all of us by the media is confusing and overwhelming. As I am typing this paragraph, I am listening to a nationally syndicated morning television program and the anchor person is interviewing a woman who has successfully lost over 50 pounds [maybe more] and is sharing her method of achieving success. One of her statements is that she exercises 3 hours per day. Now let's get real! Who has 3 hours per day to exercise? Mike and I are both professional personal fitness trainers, and WE DON'T have 3 hours per day to exercise, and we both work in a gym every day! In fact, one of the important concepts of Mike Horn's system is the 30-minute workout. The intensity and manageability, and the extraordinary SYNERGY of doing ALL of the components of the Mike Horn System SIMULTANEOUSLY make the accomplishment of a daily 30-minute exercise session extremely effective and practical.

One of the problems contributing to obesity is the mountain of incomplete or just plain WRONG information. The Mike Horn system works, for just about 100% of the people who follow the plan exactly. The reasons that people do not begin or quit the plan before success more fully explain the problem. There are cultural, sociological, biological, psychological, and financial issues that influence and even govern our perception, decisions, and beliefs. Brother Lonnie Miller, a noted Bible scholar and Director of a Drug and Alcohol Rehabilitation Center, the Mission of Hope, for over 40 years, has an interesting opinion about this cultural phenomenon. He states that many people will not embrace Christianity because they will not let go of their sin. If their sin is drinking alcohol, using drugs, coveting money, sex outside of marriage, the gay lifestyle, or not forgiving those who have wronged you, people cling to that which gives them comfort. The Bible clearly states that all of these behaviors are wrong, so many people choose NOT to follow Biblical principles in their every day life, and do not wish to associate with a group of people who openly embrace living by Biblical principles.

I see a similar response toward food demonstrated by our population. An example of this would be our social attitude concerning food. Sugar and alcohol are billion dollar industries, accounting for a major segment of the National and global gross national product, [GNP]. This has been true for 3 or 4 centuries, and may have been a contributing factor in the fight for Independence from Britain in the 1700's. The authors of our school system's selected history books would have school children believe that the War for Independence was fought, among other things, because of an unfair tax on tea. Now do you think for one minute that the American colonists would pick up rifles to keep their tea? Tea is certainly important to the English, and the people in China and Japan, but not here in the USA. Now, molasses [sugar] and whiskey is another matter! The history books mention, almost as an afterthought that at the same time as the celebrated Boston Tea Party, the American colonists were also upset about the Molasses and Whiskey Act, and the considerable tax levied against the entrepreneur colonists for the importation and sale of these extremely profitable commodities that are extremely important to the American population and economy. As Brother Miller states, "you worship where you spend your money and your time!" How much money and time do you think the average American citizen spends purchasing and consuming sugar [candy, donuts, cakes, pastry, ice cream, pies, soft drinks, and etc.]? What about beer, wine, and whiskey? BIG BUSINESS and highly addictive! How many businesses depend in part or entirely on the revenue from alcohol and sugar? How many stores, restaurants, bars and taverns, and factories are based on sales of these two products? Many people are not ready to address this issue, or even consider removing these foods from their daily consumption. So, this whole issue is complicated. This book is a plan that will work, whether you admit the truth of these statements or not. Mike and I both hope that you will follow these steps and gain much success in this plan.

Parent, Remington and Fischer are a team of Medical Doctors and a Psychologist who authored a book a few years ago, titled HOW TO RE-SET YOUR FAT THERMOSTAT.

This book explains the function of an organ called the hypothalamus that exists within your brain that is part of your autonomic nervous system. This organ governs automatic functions of your body, such as breathing, your heartbeat, your sleep patterns, your sex drive, and your appetite for food. If you took a new job that required you to work all night and sleep all day, and you were accustomed to working all day and sleeping all night, then this change would be difficult, especially in the beginning. You would have to go to work at 11:00 p.m., work all night until 8:00 a.m., go home, and by 10:00 or 11:00 o'clock a.m., you would be exhausted and fall asleep by 12:00 noon, sleep until 8:00 p.m., wake up, prepare for another night's work, and go to work again at 11:00 p.m., work all night until 8:00 a.m., and repeat the cycle again. From personal experience, I can tell you that for the first 3 or 4 weeks you will be tired, disoriented, confused, and irritable.

Changing your eating habits and rhythms will be a similar process. As you proceed with this diet, you will weaken the compulsive and addictive quality of your desire for certain flavors, AND you will have replaced some of those desired flavors with new and subtle flavors. These new flavors will be chosen not just for the comforting quality of the food, but also for the nutritional value and health benefits of these new foods. As you begin this process, your appetite will become more mature and sophisticated, and you will grow out of the infantile and self-destructive manner of eating and living that has contributed to the excess body fat that is making you miserable.

CHAPTER **2**

THE WORST KEPT SECRET

Who better understands how to safely and quickly lose body fat than a professional in a field where losing body fat, WITHOUT LOSING HEALTH, STRENGTH, ENERGY, OR SANITY is absolutely imperative and necessary? In this profession, if you don't lose body fat, you don't get paid, and quite often, the more fat you lose, the more you do get paid!

We are not talking about fashion models, actors, physicians or astronauts, but professional athletes. And where do the greatest and most successful professional athletes turn when they want to shed unwanted fat without losing muscle, strength, endurance, and energy? Professional bodybuilders! Charles Atlas, Joe Weider, Ben Weider, Jack LaLane, Vince Gironda, and many others have made history and careers of teaching others how to become lean and trim, without endangering their health or losing strength.

We are talking about BODYBUILDERS! Of course bodybuilders become huge, even freakish in muscle size and strength, but that is only ½ of the equation. If you wanted to become much stronger, you could follow the training regimen of Vasiliy Alekseyev the famed Russian Olympic weight lifter, or you could follow the training regimen of Arnold Schwarzenegger.

Both methods would make you super strong in the safest and shortest amount of time, but which athlete would you want to LOOK LIKE?

When Sylvester Stallone wanted to beef up and trim down for his Rocky and Rambo film roles, which regimen was closer to what he did to achieve his fat losing endeavor?

One-half of what every successful bodybuilder MUST ACCOMPLISH is lose a substantial amount of the fat stored on their bodies. A body builder that gets huge without losing substantial body fat looks a lot like Jabba the Hut from the movie, "Return of the Jedi", and does not place very high in the final pose down of a bodybuilding competition. What if you learned how to do just the fat-burning part of the equation? Without getting huge, freakish muscles [incidentally, good luck in the huge freaky muscles part of the equation- you will find that getting huge takes DECADES- the losing fat part takes 90 days.]

This book will give you secret information that excellent bodybuilders have known for decades and is not found in any other diet book. This information is NOT closely-guarded at all, in fact bodybuilders have been telling anybody who would listen for YEARS, but very few people take bodybuilders seriously, [which says more about internal psychological issues within skeptics than we can talk about here], and the only people who give bodybuilders much deserved credibility are other bodybuilders and the few people who have tried their methods, and succeeded, wildly and happily.

So, open your mind, take a deep breath, and see for yourself, you have nothing to lose but pounds of ugly fat.

Science = 4. Any activity that appears to require study and method.
5. Knowledge; especially knowledge gained through experience.
[From Middle English-knowledge, learning, French and Latin scientia, from sciens, present participle scire, to know.]

Empirical = 1. Relying upon or derived from observation or experiment.
[The American Heritage Dictionary of the English Language.]

CHAPTER 3

SECRETS OF A BODY BUILDER
THE MIKE HORN SYSTEM

I Corinthians 3:16

**"Know ye not that ye are the temple of God, and that the spirit
of God dwelleth in you?"**

I Corinthians 3:17

**" If any man defiles the temple of God, him shall God destroy;
for the temple of God is holy, which temple ye are."**

This is an outline for a book on Exercise and Diet, collaboration with Mike Horn and Rick Hoadley. Mike Horn is a champion body builder. His professional achievements include:

- Two-time Mr. Alabama
- Third place in the TEAM UNIVERSE [drug-free] Bodybuilding Competition
- Second place in the NORTH AMERICAN CHAMPIONSHIPS
- First place in the JUNIOR USA COMPETITION
- 4 National Professional Certifications as Professional Personal Trainer
- One certification in Nutrition
- AFAA-NESTA-IFPA-NESTA [American Federation of Aerobics Association-National Endurance and Sports Trainers Association (Fitness & Nutrition) –International Fitness Professional Association]
- World Champion Drug Free Bench Press Record holder
- Mike Horn is an extremely knowledgeable Professional Weight Trainer with over 30 years experience training Professional and College athletes, regular clients and many sports/injury and rehabilitation clients.

Rick Hoadley is an 8th degree black belt, and one of the founders of the United States Tae Kwon Do Alliance/International Tae Kwon Do Alliance, and has trained over a dozen professional Tae Kwon Do instructors who own and operate commercial martial arts training centers in four states and has taught professionally for 35 years. Hoadley has written and published several articles and professional manuals, and copyrighted a Tae Kwon Do Instructor's Manual that pioneered a University of West Florida study [first in the Martial Arts Profession] that scientifically documented improvement in self-esteem, grades, and social competence, [Professor William C. Martin, Ph.D. - principal researcher]

This book is the result of Hoadley's recent association with Mike, and at Mike's encouragement, became certified as a Personal Fitness Trainer with the NATIONAL ENDURANCE and SPORTS TRAINERS ASSOCIATION, (NESTA) and began Professional Training at Mike's gym, PERSONAL TRAINING AND NUTRITION in Mobile, Alabama. As Hoadley became familiar with Mike Horn's sometimes radical, always effective, approach to exercise and diet, the book slowly evolved.

The value of this book is the condensed and streamlined plan of action that is presented to the reader. This book will quickly help the reader adopt and adapt a do-able and workable plan for menus, exercise routines and schedules that will eliminate reading and comprehending hundreds of books, articles, and seminars, and benefiting from decades of trial and error experimentation that is part of any successful plan or strategy.

There is an epidemic in our country today. Obesity and related diseases are affecting 50% of the population and 100% of us indirectly, through out of control health care costs and massively reduced productivity. When presidential candidates speak about health care and acknowledge that obesity and poor health are primary reasons for the health care crisis in our country, you know that the majority of the population is concerned about this issue. William Dufty writes in his landmark book, SUGAR BLUES, that all of the industrialized nations that have diets largely inundated with processed foods, sugar, refined flour [from wheat and corn] and fried foods, are stricken with heart disease, cancer, strokes, diabetes, and certain types of mental illness [depression]. Depending which study you quote, 100 years ago the average U.S. citizen consumed 4 pounds of sugar PER YEAR, and by 1970, consumption had risen to over 140 pounds PER YEAR! Countries that have more primitive 'natural' diets experience these physical maladies rarely. You can argue exact statistics all you want, but the truth is; diet is a HUGE problem.

The 2nd phase of this nation-wide [world-wide?] affliction is a significant decrease in exercise. The modern age has brought 'modern conveniences', but the net effect of all these labor and time saving devices is that modern man [and woman] exercises dangerously less than the generation of 100 years ago. Easily over ½ of the population does not know how to exercise and they do not know how to begin or maintain a 'sensible' [insert workable or do-able and effective] exercise routine or lifestyle.

The 3rd part of this equation is that modern man has lost his spiritual center. In the past, religion contributed to the moral basis of our nation. Schools that were CREATED by the church, in one form or another, educated all of the authors of the Declaration of Independence and the Constitution. Most of these learned and pro-active men were GRADUATES of actual seminary schools, and acceptance of a moral code that was not centered on hedonistic pleasure or personal gain but on what the word of God was interpreted, and basically that was the Greater Good, compassion for your fellow man, helping the poor, forgiveness, doing God's work. When we decided that God was dead and took the Bible and prayer out of the public school system things accelerated to Hell in the familiar old hand basket.

This book is a simple answer to some very complex problems. Like many successful systems, much of the formulas in this book are presented in a trinity, for simplicity that promotes easy memorization and manageability. Obviously, most individuals may have some variable in their body chemistry, lifestyle, or sport that may require information purposely NOT include in this volume, but to get started and make real progress in losing weight [losing fat], gaining muscle, improving your general health, strength, flexibility, endurance, coordination, confidence, self-esteem, and just ole joy of being alive, read on.

For a basic encyclopedia of nutrition, you cannot do better than to read Barry Sear's 3 books, ENTER THE ZONE, MASTERING THE ZONE, and THE ANTI-INFLAMMATORY ZONE. [SUGAR-BUSTERS is the 'special-ed' version of the Zone] In one of my many conversations with Mike Horn, he once confided to me " of all the diets out there, the Zone diet makes more sense and is healthier than all the others. The problem is that to achieve success with the Zone diet, [lose more than 20# in 90 days] you have to follow the plan for 12 months, and NONE of my potential or current clients will stick with a regimen for that long to achieve their weight – loss goals. So I have modified the body-builder's competition diet to kick-start the client weight-loss and exercise program, because quick results is a great motivator for people trying to begin the difficult process of losing weight and improving their health."

One of the benefits of the plan that this book will present to you is that you will learn how to begin a diet that will immediately produce results, and you will slowly expand your knowledge [and menu] to develop a lifestyle that includes a very healthy and sensible diet, one that you can maintain for the rest of your life.

The science of the infinite diet books on the market is argued by the experts back and forth, but the bottom line is this: how much credibility does a so-called expert possess when he is a fat slob? He could be a graduate of John Hopkins Medical School but if he is overweight how much does he really know? Think about it? If a physician truly understood nutrition and health, would he or she be too fat? Would a doctor choose to be unhealthy and unattractive by allowing himself to be more than 20% body fat? And how much can you learn from someone who is blessed by a metabolism that allows him or her to consume Hershey bars and Dunkin Donuts and maintain a 12% body fat composition? This book is written by two individuals who have paid their dues in different worlds of physical training, Bodybuilding and Martial arts, and have paid attention for over 30 years to a plethora of World class experts on the subjects of strength training, aerobic exercise, bodybuilding, power lifting, flexibility training, Taekwondo, Jujutsu, Full contact Karate, and all aspects of nutritional application.

Mike Horn is an example of a serious body builder who has great insight to the challenges of the average person [many of his clients are, after all, average] as well as the professional athlete or post- surgery- rehab client, which many of his clients are. The lessons to be learned from one who has the knowledge and accomplishments of Mike Horn are extremely valuable to those interested in changing body fat composition and gaining muscle, or improving athletic performance or quality of life.

One of the basic problems facing anyone interested in losing weight [we really mean losing body-fat] is which diet to follow? The media overwhelms us with hundreds of plans and books. All claim to promote the latest breakthrough in nutritional science. This book will get you started and within 3-6 months, you can make real progress [lose body-fat] and gain enough EMPIRICAL knowledge and experience to intelligently sift through the almost infinite barrage of information, much of it meaningless, irrelevant, or simply wrong and untrue, and develop your own eating plan, for the rest of your life.

The science presented in Barry Sear's books is undeniable. The results enjoyed by successful bodybuilders for decades are undeniable. Science changes day by day or at least our explanation for observations of events in the body's daily metabolism changes as new information becomes available and understood. We have been bamboozled by so called experts and doctors that have diplomas but no authentic knowledge of how to eat. [Why would you listen to a doctor or dietician with a body-fat % over 19 %? If a physician truly knew how to lose weight, would he choose to be overweight?] The food pyramid is a joke. Our country has been tricked into this low-fat craze, and the incidence of obesity has more than doubled. Some of human metabolism is very similar to the metabolism of other mammals. Farmers have known for hundreds of years that the way to make cows fat is feed them grain. Bread, cereal, corn chips, are all grain products that when consumed in excess, cause almost immediate fat gain. Meat is not the enemy. Low fat is not the answer. The problem is the wrong type of carbohydrate, and/or carbohydrate eaten in too large of a quantity in a meal, or eaten without the essential insulin-stabilizing effect of the correct volume of protein in the same meal. None of this is addressed adequately by any eating plan except for The Zone Diet, or the diet used by hundreds of successful bodybuilders for decades.

Carbohydrates are not the problem, totally. A carbohydrate is food sources, [usually a fruit, vegetable, or grain] which contains starch, or sugar, vitamins and minerals and fiber, and are the primary source of food that provides glucose for the brain and energy for the muscles.
One of the important things I learned from Mike, [and I was able to experiment and confirm this empirically], is that some aspects of the bodybuilder's diet and exercise regimen are not formally recognized by the medical establishment, yet for whatever yet to be published explanation, these things work!

A case in point; according to Barry Sear's three books, a sweet potato is an UNFAVORABLE CARBOHYDRATE, and should account for one block (serving) of carb per meal, [1/3 or ¼ cup], and should only be eaten in extreme moderation else the insulin response from such a starchy sugary carbohydrate spike insulin levels and put your metabolism into fat-storing mode. I have tremendous respect for Barry Sears, his body of work, and the common sense and sophisticated science he so clearly presents in his books. According to Sears, if the meal you consume contains too much volume of carbohydrate or protein, or even a carb that is too high on the glycemic index, your pancreas will be stimulated and your body will produce too much insulin too rapidly, and when insulin levels are too high, insulin is a chemical message to your muscles to STORE fat. You could be running a marathon, and if your insulin levels are out of balance for your metabolism, you can only store fat, not burn it. Sears presents a very clear picture of how your pancreas responds to the food you eat. If your meal is too much volume of carbohydrate or protein for your muscle mass and activity level to burn and utilize at the time you eat, then your body will store the digested food, as fat. If your meal is the appropriate volume and type of carbohydrate, then you are THERMOGENIC, and you burn fat, and cannot store it. I believe that the science that Sears presents is accurate, but I also know that when I follow Mike's diet, I eat 2-3 WHOLE sweet potatoes daily and burn fat steadily, maintain a constant and steady supply of glucose to my brain, build muscle and strength, and enjoy a very high level of energy to perform my daily activities. I know that Barry Sears presents the science necessary to calculate lean muscle mass, daily activity level intensity, grams of protein, carbohydrate, and fat necessary to fuel the brain and muscles, rebuild and maintain tissue, and provide a steady supply of energy for the individual. I learned to calculate these variables accurately and achieved success in changing my body fat % and energy levels in a positive direction, and I know that Sears is on target with his information.

But I cannot explain why when I follow Mike's diet that his diet works more efficiently: much, much, more efficiently! I cannot explain why when I follow Mike's diet plan, that sweet potatoes are an EXCELLENT source of energy for me? Completely contrary to everything I have learned by reading Sear's books, and many other nutritional texts. I have learned that when I eat sweet potatoes, with appropriate volumes of protein such as tuna, chicken or lean beef, I burn fat and build muscle, and enjoy high levels of steady energy and mental clarity. I can only conclude, as Mike says, that bodybuilders collectively, know things about burning fat and building muscle that medical science has not yet published. I know, from actual trial and error, that when I follow Mike's diet, I burn fat, build muscle, gain strength, enjoy high levels of energy, and FEEL GREAT!

I know that I am hypoglycemic, and if I eat a carbohydrate without appropriate volume of protein and fat at the same meal, my insulin levels will rise, and my blood sugar level will plummet, and I will experience hunger, lightheaded dizzy sensations, depression and difficulty thinking clearly. I have learned this by reading many books; LOW BLOOD SUGAR AND YOU, (Carlton Frederick), Barry Sear's three books, ENTER THE ZONE, MASTERING THE ZONE, THE ANTI-INFLAMMATORY ZONE, SUGAR BLUES (William Dufty), and the books written by David Atkins. I have experimented with the suggestions presented by these authors and I know from repeated experiments that when I ingest sugar, and any food that is 'unfavorable' or high on the glycemic index, I will experience very unpleasant consequences, including fat gain. I don't need one more experience ingesting unfavorable carbs to know absolutely, that I will suffer a negative response to this type and amount of these carbs.

But I cannot explain why when I follow Mike's suggestions in diet, that sweet potatoes are an EXCELLENT source of energy for me. I cannot explain why when I eat sweet potato, tuna, or chicken, or in the later stages of the eating plan, lean beef with the sweet potato, I do not store fat, I burn fat, I build muscle, and I enjoy very high levels of energy.

I can only conclude, as Mike says, that bodybuilder's collectively, know things about burning fat and building muscle, that medical science has not yet published. All I know is, that regardless of what I have read, when I follow the eating plan this book will give you, I burn fat, gain muscle and strength, have great levels of energy, and FEEL GREAT!

Another aspect of this kick-start competitor's diet that is extremely interesting is the amount of food that you and I will consume as the weeks of adhering to the plan pass. The more strictly I follow the diet, the more food I want to eat, and the leaner I become. The self-esteem that accompanies this change in your metabolism and your decreasing body-fat % is irresistible and powerful. The more success I achieve, the stronger my resolve becomes. Every time I cheat on the diet, the more determined I become as I again begin the diet, the very next meal an opportunity to be successful, again. I know from reading Sear's books that it is possible to calculate EXACTLY, to the gram, the amount of protein, fat, and carbohydrate that my lean muscle mass and activity level demand to maintain adequate tissue repair and energy levels. Yet, as I follow the diet, somewhere between the 5th and 6th week, I find that I am eating constantly, 10-12 meals per day, yet I slowly become leaner and more muscular. It is as if my body, my stomach and my brain, know instinctively, perfectly, exactly how much protein and carbohydrate and fat my body needs, hour by hour. Better than any human measurement or calculation, becoming one with the diet brings my consciousness in tune with the precise amounts of nutrients and schedules for eating my brain and body need. Did God not create a miracle when He created our body and our brain? "THE DIET" is known as 'eating clean', body-builder's slang for the purification process of combining extremely scientific and effective exercise and eating schedules and routines so that we do become ' purified '. As the body-builder [and you] become more accustomed to "THE DIET', you become more motivated to continue 'THE DIET".

Protein is one of the most essential components of nutrition, and for an endeavor as difficult as losing body fat adequate daily (hourly) amounts of protein are absolutely mandatory. The immune system is 90 % protein, and how many human diseases and maladies are related to an inadequate immune system? PROTEIN POWER, (Michael and Dana Eades) is another very well written and researched book that will give the reader background on correct and accurate information about human nutrition, and the authors are very adamant about the absolute necessity of adequate amounts of quality protein. One of the variables in the successful formula of losing body-fat and maintaining health is BUILDING MUSCLE. Forget any thoughts like 'I don't want to look like a bodybuilder- I just want to get toned'. So many people say this when they first come to the gym, and this statement exposes extremely flawed thinking, a comment based on zero information and serious fallacy. IF you trained like a maniac, like Mike Horn or Arnold Schwarznegger or the current Mr. Olympia, Ronny Coleman, and were blessed with PERFECT genetics, and followed exactly the nutritional and exercise guidelines determined by any of these three experts in bodybuilding, you might possibly gain 8-10 # of muscle in ONE YEAR- 12 MONTHS- 365 DAYS of training harder than anything you have attempted in your life! Do you think that a gain of 8# of muscle in 12 months will be a big deal in your appearance? You are kidding yourself if you think that by lifting weights you are going to transform yourself into an Arnold look-alike in a year. This book is not about kidding yourself, but a serious guide for quickly and expertly getting you started in transforming you from where are now in health, appearance, body-fat %, strength and energy to your desired goal of health, appearance, body-fat %, strength and energy. The reason you MUST learn how to build muscle is that unless you increase or maintain the performance of your muscles, you will LOSE the ability of your muscles to perform, and part of this atrophy will be that your muscles will not burn fat as efficiently as when you were younger. One of the reasons that Jack LaLane has become an icon in the fitness profession is that even as he has gotten older in years, his health, strength, and energy has become legendary, far beyond what a man decades younger than Jack might be capable of performing. This is because Jack LaLane has for most of his life eaten and exercised in a very scientific and efficient manner.

Mike used a very simple analogy to explain how muscle building factors in the weight loss equation. Imagine you bought a car, and drove it without an oil change or adding oil for 200,000 miles, only filling the gas tank as needed. Obviously, the auto would develop very serious mechanical problems, probably long before 200,000 miles were traveled.

If you attempt to burn fat only by performing aerobic exercise you are in effect stripping fluid from the muscle, similar to driving a car and never adding oil. The fluid you strip from the muscle is excreted in perspiration when you perform aerobic exercise. Anaerobic exercise is how you build muscle, similar to adding oil to the engine of your auto. Lifting weights is adding fluid to the muscle, and the fluid you add is blood when you 'pump' the muscle.

When you develop a muscle to become stronger, you train the muscle to do more work in less time, and one of the by-products of this training is that your muscles will become conditioned to access energy sources within the body, among these energy sources, creatine phosphate, glycogen, and BODY FAT. So, if you do not build the muscle, you will slowly lose your body's ability to burn fat efficiently. The effect of this program is to slowly fine-tune your metabolism to easily and frequently access body-fat as an energy source and to maintain a normal routine of 'clean-eating' and effective exercise.

Without adequate amounts of protein, your muscles cannot repair and grow new tissue, and then the muscles cannot become stronger, and one of the desired by-products of increasing strength is improving the muscle's ability to burn fat. So lots of protein is mandatory, and this plan will develop your metabolism so that your hunger drive will be an uncannily accurate barometer of how much protein [and carbohydrate and fat] your muscles need. The chapters on exercise will explain in much more detail about how exercise will complete the synergy of the Mike Horn system.

Fat is the next component in the diet. Man can live without carbohydrates, Eskimos have done this for millenniums, and until processed foods were introduced to the Eskimo population, had very little of our modern diseases.

But man cannot live without fat in the diet. Fat is essential for energy, health, and even survival. Fat is an excellent energy source, but when we are losing body fat, fat becomes a catalyst that slows the metabolism and we want to learn to safely learn to limit the total amount of fat we eat for a specified length of time, and learn how to eat healthy amounts and types of fat, and as we achieve our goals of attaining leaner body-fat % and learning to re-introduce fat into our diet in a manner that will benefit our health without causing unwanted fat gains.

In the first few weeks of this diet, we will survive on the fat found only in tuna, salmon and broiled chicken in the diet, and alternate chicken and fish for the next few weeks. Finally, we will reach the stage of the diet where we will alternate lean beef, chicken, and fish with sweet potato, oatmeal, rice, green salads, green high-fiber vegetables, and ZERO sugar, fruit, oils and fats except for the fish and specified uncooked oils. After 3 months [12 grueling weeks], you will be advised how to slowly introduce dairy products, fruit, and specified fat sources.

One of the concepts that Mike and I both agreed upon is the danger of sugar. The attitude of many dieticians and so-called experts is schizophrenic. Recently the 'TODAY' program featured one of these 'experts' discuss children's breakfast cereal and her 'recommendation' was that parents allow ' no more than 6 grams of sugar per serving' for their children. Anybody that endorses 6 grams of sugar per serving for anyone is out of their mind, and should be told to shut up and sit down. If you are tired of being overweight [we really mean too fat], then wake up and realize that sugar is NOT your friend, any more than heroin, cocaine, or cigarettes. Sugar will only raise your insulin levels, and defeat your attempt at losing body fat, building muscle, and achieving health. White sugar, brown sugar, honey, high fructose corn syrup, dextrose, and maltin: All of these substances are empty calories and will sabotage your exercise and diet efforts.

Alcohol is another saboteur and drinking alcohol, especially during the 1st 3 months, is denial. No athletes who are serious and successful, drink while they are in training, and if you wish to conquer this overweight [we really mean FAT] issue, then bite the bullet and QUIT drinking, for at least the 1st 90 days. If you cannot fathom ceasing drinking alcohol for 90 days, perhaps you have more at issue than just being overweight [too fat]. Alcohol is a refined carbohydrate, actually sugar, and one of the effects of consuming additional sugar is to complicate the insulin response in your body. In the book of Deuteronomy 21:20,

> ***"And they shall say unto the elders of his city, this our son is stubborn***
> ***and rebellious, he will not obey our voice, he is a glutton and a drunkard."***

The sins of gluttony and drunkenness are mentioned in the same verse. Apparently this problem has been around for a long time, and even the ancient Jews knew they were both serious health and social issues, and even they weren't sure which was worse, being an alcoholic or obese.

Again, this diet is not for anyone who is NOT serious about losing body fat, and is a plan that will get positive results, quickly and safely. You will make sacrifice, but not unbearable and not for long. What you will attain in the 1st 90 days will be wonderful even if the amount of fat loss you achieve is not your complete goal, what fat loss you do achieve will be a great start, and as you expand the diet, you will continue to exercise and eat in a disciplined and planned schedule, you can continue to lose body fat, although not as quickly as in the 1st 90 days.

CHAPTER 4

REALITY VERSUS PUBLISHED AND PRINTED INFORMATION-SCIENCE?

I spent a year working at Mike Horn's gym and I would ask questions daily about diet and training. I was very impressed with Barry Sear's book, ENTER THE ZONE, and had modified my diet enough that I was able to lower my body-fat % from 21% to 17% in 90 days. I learned about the science of controlling hormones [insulin and glucagons] through content and portion size, monitoring activity level, frequency of meals, and learning my lean muscle mass protein requirements, and how to effectively proportion grams of carbohydrate to grams of protein and grams of fat. I was confident in my newfound knowledge and new lean and trim body, and very grateful for my great increase in energy throughout the day.

I was never skeptical of anything Mike said to me, but I was very secure and confident in my own experience and successful results I achieved following Barry Sear's suggestions from his books. One recurring comment that Mike often shared was "bodybuilder's have known this fact for years!" I was certainly very interested in what Mike said, and you have to see Mike in person to truly understand my point. Mike is 6 feet tall and 260 # of giant wedge-shaped rock-hard muscle. According to Mike, there are much bigger bodybuilders, Ronny Coleman [8 time Mr. Olympia] is one of the athlete's that Mike admires greatly, but I have never had the opportunity to train and pick the brain of anyone with Mike's practical knowledge in my life. Regardless of how many bodybuilders are bigger or more advanced than Mike, he is very accomplished in achieving personal goals. Mike looks like a bodybuilder. He has the same muscles as you and me; his are just much, much larger, perfectly shaped for maximum strength, and very visible underneath his skin. Mike hovers at 8%-10% body-fat year round, and for his competitions, drops down to 2%-4% body-fat %. Truly a remarkable human being, especially when you realize he has developed his size and physique and metabolism by learning his profession expertly, and decades of hard work. His father and brother are very close to Mike, and they are very normal in stature. Mike is not gifted with any special genetics for size or metabolism, but has literally transformed himself and his lovely wife, Jan, [Ms. Alabama] into extremely healthy, strong, fit, and competitive athletes.

So I listened to Mike, and slowly I became very curious to find how this all worked, empirically. This chapter is a simple plan that will take you, dear reader, on a journey that is exciting, healthy, and may surprise you with positive improvements in your metabolism, body-fat %, appearance, strength, and energy level.

Mike and I have discussed the issue of denial at great length. We agree on one stipulation before you will succeed with this or any other diet, and that is that you are READY to do anything to finally shed those unwanted pounds. If you absolutely will not exercise, will not STOP EATING CERTAIN FOODS, then you will NOT succeed, and you might as well resign yourself to living the rest of your life as a fat slob. You may occasionally lose weight, [usually muscle tissue and fluid] and gain back more body fat and slowly get fatter and older, and more miserable and resigned to the hopelessness of your plight. But, IF you can be open-minded, you will learn much about yourself, and the human species.

Are you a Homo sapiens, a thinking human being? Or are you a helpless, weak, Pillsbury doughboy completely controlled by your insatiable desire for the addictive pleasure of your taste buds? A mindless slave, which is blindly nursing on the next high-fat sugary treat? Unaware of how tiny your comfort zone is, automatically accepting the overwhelming volume of bread, sugar and alcohol that is a cultural imperative in our society.

Are you really so lazy and stupid that you will NOT even experiment by making a small change in your daily routine to become healthier and less repulsive looking? Or do you enjoy resembling a walrus or elephant seal?

God designed this world to make the taste of food a pleasure for mankind, not the sole purpose of eating. We eat to rebuild our bodies and give us energy, and eat to live, [a healthy life]; we should NOT LIVE TO EAT!

Some monkeys held in captivity exhibit constant, compulsive, obsessive masturbation because of some developmental glitch associated with isolation and prolonged captivity. If a human was a slave to sexual pleasure, to the point of threatening his health and becoming a visible social outcast, we would all recognize the inappropriate nature of that person.

But because food is such a universal source of comfort, we give fat people a very insincere pass. In the presence of an overweight friend or family member, we insist that 'it is what is inside a person that counts, not their appearance', while privately, we make fun of such individuals. Whether it was Jackie Gleason, John Belushi, or Chris Farley, fat people are funny, not sexy, and not to be taken seriously. Subconsciously, we acknowledge that this obese individual is infantile, a huge weak, soft baby, not someone capable of strength, self-control, or endurance.

But when we look in the mirror, what do we see? Anorexics see someone that is seriously fat, incapable of processing the visual reality staring back at them in the mirror. Similarly, fat people develop a kind of survival/denial mentality and perception. What kind of self-loathing or hidden anger or depression is fueled by the plague of 20 or more unwanted pounds of lumpy, dimpled, jiggly rolls of flabby fat?

Very few people would pursue healthy eating, and a lifestyle of vigorous exercise without the bonus blessing of appearing svelte, sexy, energetic, and virile and strong, all attributes that boost our self-esteem and trigger powerful psychological responses within all of us, and elevate inter-personal and social status for the trim, rugged, lean –looking individual. So looks do count… at least part of the total equation.

"THE DIET" which you are about to be introduced works! You can listen to the daily news show barrage of the latest diet debate, and become more and more confused by the latest edition of so-called experts, or you can demonstrate some courage, resolve, and initiative and DO this for 90 days. You will learn much about whom you are and what makes you tick, as well as what makes you fat and thin.

If you are so attached to the parts of your belief system that you cannot accept the fact that if you want to change your appearance and body weight, you will first have to change your behavior, which means you will have to change what you eat, and learn to exercise. If you are unwilling to do this, then you are doomed to get more of what you have now, and you will be fatter than you want to be, even gain more fat, and slowly erode your health because you don't have a clue how to maintain a lifestyle that is good for you.

One of the most perplexing aspects of training clients to become more fit, leaner, and stronger is the observing and recognizing the denial demonstrated denial by many clients. Almost like an alcoholic or drug addict denying the chaos that using drugs and alcohol is adding to their life, people that are troubled by too much fat are in total denial. A typical example might be my conversation with my most recent potential client. During the last 2 months, we have discussed an initial trial exercise session to determine if she would wish to begin a month of personal training sessions. It has not happened yet, apparently the only time she has to exercise is Saturday afternoon, and because my schedule is full for about 60 hours per week, and I am reluctant to add one more client to an already overbooked schedule. Once again, priorities! This may be the single most important point of the Mike Horn system; that to begin losing weight [body-fat] is such a daunting task that it is self-defeating to begin a program that is not as balanced and effective as the Mike Horn system. The time, effort, sacrifices, and change required is often under-estimated. The amount of exercise necessary to burn fat is exhausting! That is one reason that athletes and farm workers sleep so well; they are very tired. If you are just learning to begin a new exercise regimen [lifestyle] then you do not want to gain fat every day, you want to burn fat, and you want to become THERMOGENIC. You will reach your goals of fat-loss much more quickly, with a MINIMUM OF EXERCISE AND EFFORT, by adhering to the directions in this system. Denial is obvious when a client who is obviously overweight, [too fat!] decides VERBALLY, to begin the Mike Horn system, and although this client agrees with the steps and principles of this system, continues to eat and not exercise just as they did before they agreed to begin the system. When you begin the Mike Horn system, several things happen simultaneously; you learn how to "tune-up" your muscles, [make the muscle capable of burning fat at optimum levels], you learn to burn fat with a minimum of TIME and EFFORT, but, most importantly, you learn how to change your diet for a few short weeks, and become thermogenic. Remember, nutrition is 90% of it! If you eat differently than this diet suggests you will slowly gain fat, perhaps as little as 1or 2 ounces per day. At the end of a week of working hard, you will have GAINED 1- 2 pounds INSTEAD OF LOSING 1-2 pounds. How disappointing! What Mike Horn is teaching all of us is this; losing fat is difficult, don't make this task more difficult. In fact, optimize and maximize your effort. Know that this diet will safely feed your muscles and brain, give you maximum energy, and quickly eliminate the foods and quantities that make you fat. The exercise component of the Mike Horn system makes the fat-loss quicker and extremely efficient. The quick progress is an important psychological component in developing and strengthening RESOLVE. As you improve your success, you validate this eating and exercise plan, and you know that you are on the right path. If you understand this whole process, begin the plan, but deny that you are NOT following the steps carefully, and then you are in denial.

Just as many men I meet who discuss self-defense or building muscle [and I am sure repairing automobile engines!] think that because they posses male genitalia, they are also experts in both of these subjects, and will argue with me endlessly about any aspect of fighting or building muscle. Likewise, this woman repeatedly mentioned to me" how fat she was", and that she "only had 10 pounds to lose." She repeatedly said that she didn't think that bread made her fat. When I replied that the current thinking I was exposed to stated that corn and bread act like sugar in most people's metabolism, she responded with "I don't agree!" Of course she doesn't agree, she wants to eat bread! Yet she is the one stating that she is 10 pounds overweight. She is searching for some way to experiment and keep what she wants to eat, and somehow figure out a way to exercise and lose weight. You CAN lose weight with any number of diets, and some will work for you, some won't. The advantage of the MIKE Horn System is that it will work, safely, in the shortest amount of time, with the least amount of suffering, almost like having surgery. You can lose weight another way, but you will spend much more time to reach your goal, and success may be extremely difficult. This system has ALREADY failed many different ways, for decades, and has been adjusted and modified repeatedly after each failure, so that the plan you are presented minimizes the variables so much that you can quickly identify what you need to correct and get back on the schedule of burning fat and building muscle. You can quickly follow this plan and achieve your goals, or you can re-invent the wheel and do endless research, figure out that Mike Horn is right, and then write your own book with very similar guidelines.

Losing body fat is difficult for trained and experienced athletes, and if all of this attention to diet and exercise is new to you, then you will experience difficulty also. Don't you want to make this feat less painful and as simple as possible? Doesn't it make sense to use a proven plan that is safer, quicker, and the most effective and efficient as possible?

You may have to give up bread, and sugar, and booze, at least takes control of how much and how often you eat the foods that make you over fat, but aren't giving up things that are destructive for you to become the new lean, trim you, worth the effort? If not, quit reading, and resign yourself to remain at the body fat % you are now. If you are ready to begin one of the most positive chapters of your life, then read on.

Another observation that will help you grasp the concept of this eating plan that makes it works: This plan works fast- faster than ANY other diet known, that is why professional body builders use this diet. This diet is safe - you will not LOSE muscle - but actually GAIN muscle while following this plan.

You are not deprived of either protein OR carbohydrate- so your muscles repair, rebuild and grow and your muscles and brain get enough food so you have plenty of energy and mental clarity to perform all your daily tasks AND add a short 30 minute burst of exercise to add to the stimulation you are giving your metabolism.

The only deprivation you will experience briefly is a big difference in the frequency and quantity of flavor that brings you pleasure. You must come to terms with WHY you eat. Again, if you are ruled ONLY by the PLEASURE that food brings to your senses, and then consider that your old habits and food choices have perverted your appetite and sense of taste. Remember, this is a TEMPORARY pause in tasting pleasurable flavors, and by completing this plan, you will accomplish several important objectives.

First, you will begin losing fat very quickly. Second, you are kick starting your metabolism, and that benefit can remain with you for a long, long time, hopefully for the rest of your life. Third, you are cleansing your body by beginning this program, and renewing and rejuvenating your mental and emotional approach and perception concerning food and eating. Just as an over-worked person goes on a vacation to rest and become refreshed, you are returning to SQUARE ONE of your mental paradigm concerning these essential bodily functions by taking a break from the destructive habits that are making you fat and miserable, and forming new habits based on positive choices that are selected for the health benefits of eating according to this plan.

Another of the most perplexing aspects of understanding the reality of "The Diet" is being in a hospital and being surrounded by 'health professionals'. Over and over I see obese health professionals and I tell myself that 'if they really knew about nutrition and exercise, they would not be so- over fat.

I was in the hospital recently for a hip replacement surgery, and I was discussing my meals with my physician and my nurse and the dietician. As I made my wishes known concerning my meals I could see the eyebrows rising all around. The choices I was making to survive on sweet potatoes, oatmeal, tuna fish, chicken, lean beef, vegetables, water, coffee, no sugar, only healthy, clean types and portions of fat; were causing alarm and concern because my choices did not co-incide with the published science that these well-meaning and concerned professionals believed to be truth. The prospect of me eating according to my plan was terrifying to these people, and they viewed the prospect of me eating a menu that was not part of the established theory as DANGEROUS!

Ask yourself, what could possibly be more dangerous than gaining fat? And while I am healing from the surgeon's incision, I must have adequate protein at all times.

Please, dear reader, do not judge this diet until you have tried it for 90 days.

CHAPTER 5

SUGAR - YOUR WORST ENEMY!

This chapter will upset you. Some readers will put this book down in disgust before they finish reading this chapter. Sad, because to finally get a grip on this too-fat/overweight problem, you must LEARN why you are fat and the woman standing next to you in line at the supermarket is NOT too fat. Or why your co-worker can eat chocolate doughnuts every morning for breakfast and is as thin as a rail. Or why you want to lose 30 #, but thank God you are not as heavy as the woman you saw at the Mall yesterday, poor thing, she must have to lose 100#!

Nutrition is a science, and the subject is complex. The current calorie/fat theory and related food pyramid is ONLY a theory, AND a theory that is obviously flawed and not a valid explanation for the reality we all observe right before our eyes.

The books written by Barry Sears [ENTER THE ZONE, MASTERING THE ZONE, THE ANTI-INFLAMMATORY ZONE] and PROTEIN POWER [Michael and Dana Eades] present the most logical answer to the perplexing question of why being too fat is such a difficult problem to understand and correct.

The answer is NOT that every fat person eats too much and exercises too little, although that is certainly part of the equation. The problem is not quite that simple, any more than stating that every single person who smokes cigarettes will die of lung cancer. Cancer does not present in every smoker. Fact! Obviously, the cancer question is complicated, and cannot be answered with a broad sweeping statement like smoking causes cancer, [although smoking DOES cause cancer, just not in every single smoker]. Being too fat is not caused by eating too much, [although eating too much IS an important part of the equation] but eating too much for YOU, your eating pattern and habits and exercise pattern and habits.

This chapter will present the most logical condensation of information science, history, and common sense that the authors can offer to shed light on this confusing subject of fatness.

According to the books mentioned at the beginning of this chapter, man was once a hunter and food gatherer. Early man survived by hunting animals, and picking berries and nuts, cutting grasses and digging up roots and vegetables, picking fruit, catching fish and birds, and taking advantage of every opportunity to eat a protein, fat, and carbohydrate, ingest vitamins and minerals, trace elements, and all the substances known and unknown that make up the smorgasbord of food that keeps a human healthy.

Best information available states that approximately 10,000 years mankind started growing and cultivating grasses, vegetables, and fruits. Grains especially, contained some protein, fat, as well as a plentiful source of needed carbohydrate, and better than fruit, vegetables, meat and fat, could be stored easily for long periods of time [especially in hot, moist climates, or freezing climates] without spoiling.

At about this same time, man also killed off most of the wild animals, certainly in certain parts of the Middle East, Europe, Asia, and more recently, North America. As these herds and populations were slowly hunted out of existence [simultaneously civilization also changed or destroyed habitat necessary for these animals], mankind replaced animal protein with much less protein-content grain. The result of this transformation was that some of the population demonstrated a severe insulin response to a large volume of carbohydrate [without adequate protein volume eaten at the same meal] and gained body fat and became afflicted with the attendant diseases that are in part CAUSED by an unfavorable insulin response, These people became fat, their basic health deteriorated as diseases such as diabetes, heart attacks, strokes, triglyceride/ cholesterol / blood problems, cancer, depression, emerged from obscurity and became epidemic.

According to PROTEIN POWER, archeologists can determine almost within 100 years which century that the population of Egypt shifted from hunting/food gathering to growing crops. The basis of this hypothesis is the evidence of tooth decay, wrinkled skin indicating obesity, evidence of heart disease and clogged arteries, and precursors of many of the maladies that afflict our modern age.

In contrast, when archeologists find bones of ancient humans with perfect teeth, massive strong skeletons and evidence of powerful muscles, the determination is that these remains belong to humans that were hunters, not farmers. Ancient farmers could not raise enough domestic animals to supply daily protein needs, and regardless of what the vegetarians will tell you, grain and vegetables cannot provide enough protein for the average humans' daily requirements. Without enough protein, muscles lose strength, size, and the ability to burn fat efficiently.

According to authors Eades and Sears, approximately 50% of the population cannot eat quantities of carbohydrate without similar volumes of protein at the same meal without responding with a rapid rise in insulin levels. 50 % of the population apparently can eat large quantities of carbohydrate with no erratic insulin response, or any other deleterious effect. So obesity and an overworked pancreas are the result of too much carbohydrate in the diet, and too little protein.

The reader can read both of the above mentioned books to gain insight to more detail of the facts of human history and biology, and this book is focused on the plan that will bring success, not a complete explanation of the scientific theory that is the reason this plan will work for you. I cannot explain to you exactly HOW the theory of electricity actually works; I just know that if you push the light switch to the "ON" position, the light will become lit. If you the reader will approach this book with a similar open-minded attitude, you will find that in 90 days you have lost body fat, become leaner, gained muscle, strength and energy, and you will have gained valuable self-knowledge about why you eat, about your comfort zone, and many other aspects of your behavior and the results of your behavior on your health and well-being.

One of the surprising features of this diet is the sheer volume of food you will eat. As your metabolism speeds up, you will be hungry more quickly, and you will eat more often than you think is 'normal'. As your metabolism speeds up, you will burn more fat than you did before, and you will have more energy, and you will become more active and do all the normal routines of the day with more intensity.

Remember, bodybuilder's uses this diet, and bodybuilders cannot afford to lose muscle mass, in fact, bodybuilders must gain muscle mass while burning fat. Even wrestlers and gymnasts will benefit from thus diet, because of the quality of the diet.

Because you are learning to limit the amount of fat in your meals, you will digest your food quickly. One of the benefits of fat in your diet is that fat digests slowly, and each gram of fat contains 9 calories, compared to 4 calories of energy per gram of protein or carbohydrate.

Another benefit of fat is flavor, and appetite satiation. If you cannot survive for 90 days without bread, spaghetti, ice cream, or chocolate or butter, than you are choosing pleasure OVER your health or achieving your goal and you will probably remain fat. You will be amazed at what you can do if you have to, once you 'put your mind to it'.

As you become more successful with this diet, you will be pleasantly surprised at how your attitude toward food changes. You will also notice how much you appreciate new foods and flavors once you attain your body fat goals and begin to expand your diet and start eating more 'normal' meals.

Another aspect of 'THE DIET' that is extremely healthy is the idea of planning your meals for the day, and EATING BEFORE YOU GET HUNGRY! If you have a healthy meal prepared ahead of time to eat, then you will not become so ravenous that you over eat, or cheat with foods that are not on the diet. If you eat a balanced meal of 4-6 ounces of quality protein and a 'good' carbohydrate, such as sweet potato, rice, or oatmeal, and a high fiber vegetable or salad, you will enjoy a 'full' feeling of eating, and keep your blood sugar/ insulin levels stable and steady. High insulin levels drive down blood sugar levels in your blood stream and you will feel hungry, lightheaded and nervous. When you eat 'clean', you will have plenty of energy; your brain will have plenty of fuel and good mental clarity. Your muscles will have adequate energy and protein for fuel and repair. When you can think clearly, and your nutritional needs are met, you can more easily focus on more meaningful activities than feeding your face. If you are exercising as prescribed in 'THE DIET', you will be more relaxed and ready for a good night's sleep at the end of the day.

You may prepare as many as 10 –12 meals per day, and put them in Tupperware containers, refrigerate and keep in a large insulated lunch box or soft vinyl cooler. If you sense your stomach growling, or hunger pangs beginning, you can eat. Gradually, you will become less obsessed with food. If every meal you eat is providing needed protein and carbohydrates, you never give your body a chance to develop intense hunger, and you will slowly begin to eat in a rhythm that is tuned to your personal nutritional needs rather than some arbitrary 'meal-time'. You will observe that at first you will become 'burnt-out' by eating certain foods over and over. But, gradually, you will become more adapted to the foods on 'THE DIET' and the stability of your hormonal system and the general sense of well being will become more attractive and important. As you begin to melt body fat and become leaner and more trim, you will slowly change your perspective from a person who is over fat because of a COMBINATION of habits that are not suited for your metabolism, food selection, and activity level; to a person who has greater AWARENESS of your own personal needs to maintain optimum health and desired body fat %.

CHAPTER **6**

THE KICK-START DIET

You have to eat breakfast every morning. Coffee and tea can be good for you, but to start the "DIET" you need to fill the muscle with fluid. Drink coffee or tea only before weight training. Caffeine stimulates the body to burn carbs as an energy source instead of burning fat as an energy source during exercise. Soda is of no value, except to satisfy cravings. For every soda you drink, double your water intake immediately after you drink the soda, coffee, of tea. Coffee, tea or soda dehydrates the muscle.

Stop eating out in restaurants for two weeks. No fast food or restaurants, because eating out in restaurants contributes to developing cravings and overeating. Fats and sugars fuel the fast food and restaurant industry, at the expense of your health. Very few people have the knowledge, resolve and discipline to eat at a restaurant without overeating, or making poor choices in selection of foods. If you can eliminate these fats, sugars, and foods from your menu, your cravings will slowly diminish.

Wake up at the same time every day, for at least the first two weeks. Take two CLA (conjugated linoleic acid) capsules and two max lean fat burners, with water within 3 minutes of waking. Within 10 minutes of waking, eat the first meal of the day.

Meal # 1 - 5 egg whites scrambled, use spray PAM in frying pan, ½ cup of oatmeal, flavor with Splenda, cinnamon, and spray butter flavor. If you are still hungry, eat more of the same foods as desired.

Eat every 3 hours, whether you are hungry or not.

Meal # 2 - One skinless, boneless chicken breast,[use any seasoning] one small round red potato, and one cup of any green vegetable, [green beans] or I cup of red beans and rice. Cook this from scratch yourself and use NO butter. Make enough for several days and store in Tupperware- add shredded chicken breast [as much as you want].

Meal # 3 - Your choice - 1 or 2 turkey burger patties with fat free cheese, measure 3/4 cup brown rice OR a protein shake – use high quality protein powder, such as High-5 or XP protein.

Meal # 4 - Baked, steamed or grilled fish, [any fish is ok to begin your program]. Wal-Mart steams tilapia- Winn-Dixie steams any fish you buy; your local grocer may do the same. Steaming at the store makes great ease and convenience to take the fish home and heat or eat without time-consuming preparation. Grilled okra, onion, and peppers are great with fish. You may eat any vegetable [2 cups] with your fish.

Meal # 5 - Your choice – a snack pack tuna- no mayo-or all natural peanut butter [no sugar or hydrogenated oil] on apple slices. Or, 2 fat-free hot dogs, with low carb ketch-up and baked chips.

When you become hungry, or for one reason or another cannot prepare one of your meals according to the "DIET" menu, you may fall back on eating a meal of tuna and a sweet potato. If you add an extra meal or two during the day, or as a midnight snack, this basic meal will nourish your metabolism and can help you resist the temptation to cheat with worse choices for food.

Drink 1 gallon of water daily. Use sugar free Tang or Kool-Aid or crystal-light.

This is the basic eating plan for the first 4 weeks.

SEVEN TOP PRIORITIES

Mike has presented 7 top priority new habits to create.

#1. Water - your water intake is critical. Most health related doctors are diagnosing problems without knowing the patient's diet. Drinking plenty of clean water also flushes your system of toxins. Free- radicals that float through your system will build up if not flushed out. Proper water intake will prevent health problems. Drinking water will also limit fluid retention that eventually leads to weight gain. The more you drink the less you retain.

#2. Food Intake - You are what you eat- garbage in- garbage out. It's that cut and dry. You should eat 4-6 meals a day. Meals do not have to be big, but you should eat some protein and carbs every meal. When you begin this plan, you must stick to it. If you have a craving for foods you know are bad for you, and you do not control the impulse to eat, then you must deal with that issue first. If you cannot stop drinking alcohol or eating sugar or chocolate for 90 days in order to begin a new life, and lose 20 #, then you are eating for reasons other than nutrition or health, in fact you are abusing food in a manner that impairs your health, and that is self-destructive at best and suicidal at worst. This means do not start a diet until you are mentally stable. Ask your family, friends, and co-workers for support. Once you get 2 weeks into the program, it gets much easier. Most of our successful clients use prayer; I don't think that is a coincidence.

#3. Exercise - Includes physical activity for 30 –60 minutes that is designed to enhance a healthy lifestyle. Weight training [anaerobic] is the most important type exercise due to the many remedies that are provided by regular training. Weight training or resistance training is the only way to actually re-shape the body.

Cardiovascular [aerobic] exercise like running, treadmill, cycling, steppers, swimming are imperative as a complement to weight training. Weight training is the foundation to aerobic training for effective weight loss. Have you ever noticed an over-weight aerobics instructor? Usually this is because the over-weight instructor does ONLY aerobic classes, and does not train anaerobically with weights.

Your body and metabolism will eventually plateau on cardio only [aerobic] exercise. Make time to do anaerobic weight training. If you are reading this and thinking, "I don't have the time", you are not prioritizing or managing your time in order of importance. Make a schedule and stick to it. Poor preparation leads to poor performance. If you fail to plan- you plan to fail. You must first take care of yourself, and then you can help others. If you are miserable, overweight, weak, you are no blessing to yourself or anyone else. If you are not happy, how can you help anyone else to become happy?

#4. Vitamins - are very important to total body function. A good multi vitamin will provide most essential vitamins, and vitamin B helps other vitamins bind to organs, bones, ligaments, tendons, muscles, etc. and multi vitamins are more effective than separate supplements. Some vitamins act as anti-oxidants, which flush out free radicals. Free radicals are chemical molecules that work like floating 'bullets 'that damage muscle and other tissue. Once a muscle is damaged by a free radical, the muscle deteriorates. Your muscles are the biggest part of your body and metabolism network. Vitamins also enhance natural energy that helps burn fat efficiently. You cannot get all or enough of essential vitamins with a normal diet and a good multi vitamin will help you complete most of your necessary metabolic functions.

#5. Minerals - are hard for the body to absorb. Take a mineral complex daily. Minerals will slowly build to a safe level and help your organs, especially your brain, muscles, and endocrine system function properly. Mineral intake can also help you resist cravings for sugar and fats, and help you maintain proper water levels in your cells.

#6. FUN! - Enjoy your life! Make your workouts fun. You should schedule regular quality time with family and friends. A healthy lifestyle is balance, and family and fun are all part of the equation

#7. Rest! Last but not least. Rest is an essential part of your body's growth process. This means burning fat, building and repairing muscle, tendons, ligaments, bones, etc. You cannot lose fat or get stronger, or relieve stress without adequate rest. This means 8 hours of sleep, preferably at one good night's sleep, and also one or more short naps. A 20-minute power nap is a great habit to recharge your batteries and make your day more enjoyable and more productive.

You can easily over train, and you will notice that even though you making great effort, you are not making the progress you hoped for. Church attendance has great benefit psychologically as well as spiritually, and all of this has direct impact on your physical and emotional and mental well-being. Prayer is an ancient tool that will cause positive changes in every thing that you do, even if you think that you do not believe in God.

When you pray daily, you will slowly develop serenity and clarity in becoming aware of how you can attain more joy in you life, and how you can be of more assistance to those around you.

Alexander Bose was the first Indian scientist [from the sub-continent] to be admitted to the Royal Academy of Science in England and he invented the Cresco graph, later named the galvanometer or lie detector. He performed experiments that documented tremendous health benefits in humans, animals, plants and even the metal in factory machines that employed regular rest periods in their daily and weekly cycles performed longer without metal fatigue and other types of mechanical malfunctions.

You need rest as an essential component in your new life style. Your brain requires several complete sleep cycles per night to organize and file new information and store in your memory banks as new knowledge. If you do not get adequate rest, you will not grow stronger muscles or experience the mental clarity necessary to perform your daily activities at optimum level, and beginning a new diet and exercise plan will be a daunting task.

As you " live " this diet, you will experience many feelings and revelations concerning the bodily sensations and pangs of hunger that fuel our appetites and our obsessions and compulsions that drive us to eat. You will understand what prisoners in concentration camps experience, or any human that suffers starvation, except you are in complete control. You are doing this VOLUNTARILY, and you are making sure that you eat the correct amount of quality protein, carbohydrate, and fat to maintain optimum health. What you are really starving is your desire, your habits, even your unconscious addiction to unhealthy foods that keep you fat. And do you want to continue to be a slave to your appetite, your sense of pleasure, to habits that you continue just because you have been eating this way for years, even though this way of eating [and living] is harming you and damaging your health in many complicated ways?

Body fat % is an important feature of total health and fitness. I wish that you the reader could sit in a conversation with Mike Horn and myself. We recently were talking about body fat %, and Mike stated that some athletes and individuals should NOT lose body fat below 12 – 15%, because those athletes NEED the fat reserves for their particular competition or sport.

I know that current science states that every pound of excess body fat adds one mile of blood vessels [capillaries] to your body, making your heart work harder to push blood through this added network of pathways. This is doubly taxing, because the fat cells are only an extra energy source, unlike muscles, they do not perform any work, fat cells do not burn energy, the fat cells ARE STORED ENERGY. Muscles support our bodies and skeletons, move our bones and limbs through space, and use carbohydrate to fuel themselves, and use protein to rebuild and repair themselves, and muscles are literally the engines of life, from our beating hearts to our running feet to our blinking eyes, our muscles are living, breathing tissue that keeps us erect, alive and moving. Fat, on the other hand, is just lumpy globs of waxy, butter –like lard, ready to melt down into appropriate compounds that can be used for energy, and that process is known as the ardous ordeal of aerobic exercise. More about that later, just remember that aerobic exercise involves effort, sweat, time, firm resolve, and a scientific plan and a regular schedule. So, the more fat you store, the more you have to sweat off, and that will involve some level of work.

But the other side of this coin of body fat % is getting the % right for you. Evander Holyfield was a guest on the Jay Leno show days before his fight with Mike Tyson. Evander was in immaculate physical condition, as always, and stated to Jay that his body fat % was 12 %. Evander looked ripped and cut, like a diamond-studded anatomy chart, and he destroyed Mike

Tyson, this was the boxing match that featured the infamous ear-biting incident, and apparently Evander was such a dynamo of strength that Tyson was overwhelmed, and in a panic of fear and rage, resorted to biting the ear of an opponent that Tyson could find no other way to stop from attacking him.

One year later, Evander Holyfield again appeared on the Jay Leno show, and this time he was scheduled to fight Riddick Bowe, and Evander claimed to be at 4% body fat. Again, Evander looked fabulous, ripped and shredded to the bone, a lean, mean, fighting machine, 8% leaner than when he fought Tyson one year earlier. An interesting note is that for the Riddick Bowe fight, Evander used former Mr. OLYMPIA, Lee Haney, as a trainer and nutritional consultant. Evander certainly looked great by body builder standards, but he was not a ball of energy and power at 4 % body fat that he was at 12%, and Evander lost the fight.

Obviously, there are more variables involved here than either Mike or I are privileged to know, but the point is this, as authors Mike and both know that body fat % is a critical vital component of total health, and most folks reading may not be interested in competing in a body building show, but everyone likes to look slim and trim, even slightly muscular, and quality of health is directly relate to body fat %.

As you approach the 90 days on the diet, you will notice some interesting changes in your body. Besides being constantly hungry, you will be leaner. You will have lost pounds of weight, but more importantly, you will have lost inches, around your waist, your thighs and buttocks, your neck and even your wrist. You know you have lost body fat when your wrist measurement is smaller than when you began the program.

Now you have come closer to your goal of desired weight and body fat %. You can now experiment with adding to your strict menu, and it would make sense to add foods that are high on the list of 'BEST" foods. This list is rated by nutrient density = vitamins, minerals, protein, fiber, healthy fats, per 100 kilocalories and how these foods rate on the glycemic index, {glycemic index measures how quickly a food raises blood glucose levels} and the anti-cancer properties of these foods.

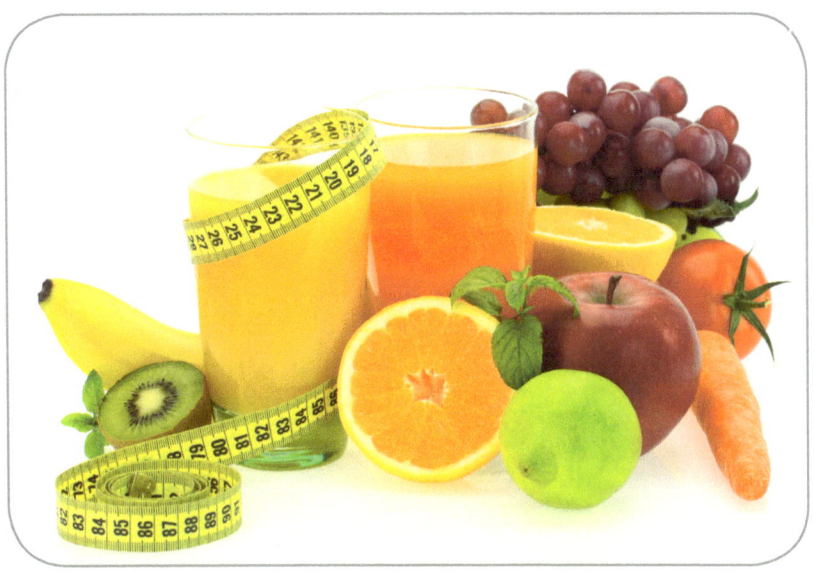

CHAPTER 8

FOODS - BEST TO WORST!

Best Foods

Oil from: fish, flax, primrose, borage, hemp, MCT, PAM, olive, sesame, and lecithin.

Protein: cod, halibut, salmon, tuna, trout, orange roughy, bass, sole, sardine, haddock. Organic liver.

Vegetables: green leafy, broccoli, cabbage, peppers, sprouts, onions, beets, tomatoes, carrots, asparagus, cauliflower, and yams [sweet potatoes]

Meat: organic liver

Fruit: oranges, apples, berries, cantaloupe, kiwi, fig, cherries, apricot, and red grapes.

Dairy: yogurt

Grains: wheat germ, brewer yeast, whole grain; barley, oats, flax, rice, rye, millet, amaranth, buckwheat, spelt wheat, and Ezekiel bread.

Beans and legumes: soybeans, garbanzo, kidney, lentils, navy beans, split peas, black-eyed peas, pinto beans, and black beans.

Herbs: spirulina, garlic, vinegar, mustard, salsa, curry, cinnamon, ginger, green tea, cayenne, stevia, and kelp.

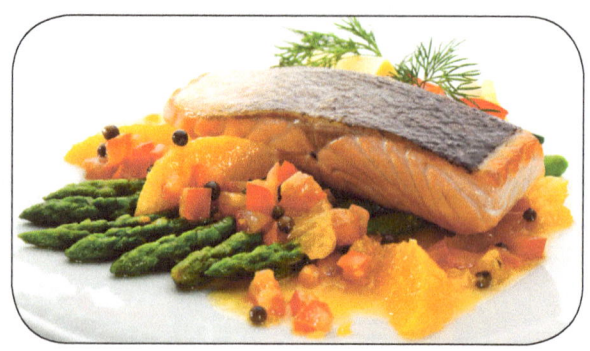

Good Foods

These foods are foods that are not the best choices but still offer high nutritional value.

Oil: canola, coconut.

Protein: turkey, chicken, lamb, liver, eggs, veal, pork, wild game, swordfish.

Vegetables: radish, celery, lima bean, zucchini, squash, lettuce, avocado, vegetable juice.

Fruits and Nuts: watermelon, grapes, honeydew, plum, banana, pineapple, papaya, walnuts, almonds, sunflower seed, and sesame seeds.

Dairy: cottage cheese, Parmesan cheese, low fat milk and cheese.

Grains and Legumes: pasta, and soy milk.

Spices: soy sauce, Worchester, Tabasco, flax seed dressing, sage, thyme, and black tea.

Fair

These foods are acceptable as part of your menu, but not your best choices for nutritional value.

Oil: soy, corn, safflower.

Protein: lobster, clams, beef, duck, shrimp, catfish.

Vegetables: olives, canned vegetables, white potatoes.

Fruit: dried fruit, raisins, dates, prunes, canned fruit.

Grain: corn chips, granola, wheat crackers, tortilla, grits.

Nuts: peanuts, peanut butter,

Dairy: regular cheese or milk.

Spices: Italian dressing, and red wine.

Treats: carob, chocolate.

All of these foods will eventually be a part of a healthy diet. You can experiment a lot once you have completed the first 90 days.

Below is a list of foods that you should consider omitting from your life. The only reason that you would eat these foods is that you are on a desert island and starving, or you are a slave to a flavor and insist on eating that particular food no matter how fat that food will make you, or how destructive to your total health that food may be. In other words, you know the truth, but you are in total denial, and do not care what the consequences are for eating that food.

Poor Choices

Commercial breakfast cereal, bacon, pizza, smoked ham, prime rib, gelatin, desserts, sweet corn, white rice or white wine, wheat, molasses, butter, beer, mayonnaise, Celtic salt, coffee, honey, fructose.

Bad Choices

Pickles, salami, bologna, sausage, hot dogs, BBQ ribs, waffles, pancakes, cookies, ice cream, blue cheese dressing.

Worst Choices

Margarine, aspartame, syrup, MSG, soda pop, diet soda, pastry, pie, doughnuts, lard, hydrogenated fat, sugar, hard liquor.

One question that we want to answer before it is asked is what about the toxic levels of mercury in fish? Won't eating so much fish poison you with mercury? Mike's answer to this question is typically insightful and to the point. "The Vikings were not worried about eating TOO much fish; they were more concerned about getting ENOUGH to eat!" Likewise when Christ fed the 5000 with 2 fishes and 5 loaves, there was no mention of mercury poisoning. The prime criticism most nutritionists have about the amount of fish that American's eat weekly or annually compared to Asian or Mediterranean peoples is that Americans don't eat ENOUGH fish! The protein in fish is less dense than the protein in beef, pork, and chicken, but it is more easily digested. It takes a greater amount of fish than other types of meat to get equal amounts of protein. Barry Sears claims in his ZONE books that in 1-ounce of meat, [28 grams], you will obtain 7 grams of usable protein. So, most meat is approximately 25% protein, and fish in less than that. Fish is an excellent source of protein because of the nature of the high-quality fats found in fish, and the big picture is that most people do not eat enough protein in their diet, and fish is a good choice because fish does not contain the dangerous types of fat that SOME cuts of meat, and most processed meat products contain. The human that eats adequate protein, carbohydrates, and healthy fats in his/her diet AND exercises intelligently will be MUCH healthier than the human who is obese or malnourished. God did design a marvelous computer and robotic piece of equipment when He made our body, and if we feed it and care for it we WILL be quite healthy.

With the same sound reasoning, we can address the issue of vegetarianism. I was a vegetarian 30 years ago, for about 18 months. I finally gave up. One of the reasons I tried to eat only plants and fruits was that I wanted to become a pacifist. When I read " THE SECRET LIFE OF PLANTS ", I realized that plants were sentient beings just like animals, that they possessed movement and response to stimulus very similar to animals, only much more slowly. If you are a vegetarian for moral issues, that is, to spare animals from being slaughtered for food, then you are deluded. It's all meat, and protein from animal sources is much higher quality than plant protein, and a higher percentage of protein than found in plants. If your reasons for being a vegetarian are based on health concerns, again, your reasoning is flawed. Eating enough protein from plant sources is a huge job, and requires hours of grazing and eating, similar to the behavior of cattle. Human beings are omnivores, and can survive on plant and animal sources, but are much stronger and healthier when fed adequate amounts of protein, and animal protein is a much more efficient method of accomplishing that objective.

Another feature of the fantasy / vegetarian school of thought is that eating meat is somehow cruel to animals. Do these fuzzy-thinking dreamers think that a wild deer checks into a retirement home when they get old? If Bambi's Mother was not shot by an evil hunter, then she would slowly starve to death as old age slowly wore her teeth down, and probably be ripped to pieces by coyotes, wolves, bears, cougars, and other predators, often helpless and still alive but too weak and slow to escape the inevitable and natural end of all prey species that have the privilege to live in the wild. All of the States in America that have a game management program now have exploding populations of healthy wild game. Deer, turkeys, ducks, geese, and a variety of game animals on this continent are experiencing an increase and stability in their numbers, not to mention the booming economic impact that hunting has on our communities. As a species, we are hunters. We are also warriors. Any human that is not fit or healthy enough to perform the physical work involved in hunting, or warfare, or at least farming and raising crops and livestock would not have survived in the days of old. Are you satisfied with your present physical condition and appearance? If so, you probably have put this book down long before you read this page. This plan is for someone who is serious about losing body fat and achieving some valuable and very personal goals. Such a person will do whatever works to become healthier as they lose body fat, even if that means they will have to learn new things. Having been a fat kid, I know how much better my life has become since my fitness and body has become ONE of the priorities of my life. I am thankful that I have enjoyed the success I have achieved, and my heart understands the misery of the poor soul who longs to be slim and attractive, but just can't make it happen. I think that genetically and instinctively we as a species feel "right "when we are healthy and energetic, and are also lean and muscular rather than rotund and out-of–breath.

Now let's get real. Nobody eats perfectly, not even world-class bodybuilders. BUT, when they cheat, they cheat rarely, and they immediately resume the diet, with more resolve and attention to the cause –and –effect of diet. At Christmas and Thanksgiving I will eat some smoked ham, and I will get fat. Not 100 # overweight, but I will develop a slight roll around my waist. One day of looking at my new found blubber will motivate me to resume the diet, and I enjoy my life much more when, a week or two later, I lose that roll, and again am at the body fat percentage that I am proud to maintain. The pleasure and reward of eating garbage, [and these poor, bad, and worse foods ARE garbage!] becomes less and less enjoyable.

The diet has become workable for me. I eat wisely more than 90 % of the time, and just like polishing off that bottle of Tequila or Scotch when I was younger and occasionally wild and crazy, I just don't enjoy indulging in alcohol any more. Likewise, I don't enjoy eating garbage anymore. I feel very good more than 90 % of the time, and I enjoy people stopping me in the grocery store and asking me where I work out, and making favorable comments about my appearance and physique, and I am not even in the same class as a bodybuilder visually. I am fit and strong and energetic, and I enjoy my body and the things I can do. You will develop similar value for the commitment and discipline you are learning to incorporate into your lifestyle. And lifestyle is the KEY word, because you are learning to live your life with STYLE! And This is NOT a style that will ever go out of fashion; health and fitness, strength and energy are eternal values that tell the world and every body you meet that you are smart and taking GOOD care of yourself. In a world where more and more people resemble Elephant seals at mating season, and life ending health problems plague almost everyone as they age, optimum health and fitness is a LOOK, a fashion statement if you will, that is appealing, attractive, and brings you unspoken respect in every social situation. If you can balance your physical appearance with a positive personality and kindness and courtesy, you will move with greater harmony in the world.

CHAPTER 9

EXERCISE IS THE OTHER 50%

This form of exercise is essential, and if you will not learn to lift weights regularly, 2-3 times per week, you will still lose weight on this diet, but you will not achieve optimum health, and slowly your muscles will deteriorate, losing tone, strength, and mass. Since muscles are the engines that burn fat, by choosing to be lazy and self-destructive and REFUSE to grow as a human being, you will find it increasingly more difficult to maintain your desired body fat %, and even more difficult to lose body fat.

Anaerobic in Greek means, 'without oxygen'. When you lift weights or perform resistance training, you work so hard for a short period that you exhaust the supply of creatine phosphate [15 second supply] or glycogen, [2 minute supply] that your muscles become temporarily unable to contract, and the cells of the muscle burn the available fuel, and the cell loses oxygen and fuel, replacing fuel with waste products such as carbon dioxide, ash, and lactic acid. They call it lactic acid for a reason: it burns!

Another benefit of anaerobic exercise is that when you approach 90% of your maximum heart rate, you become breathless, and you stimulate your pituitary gland, another gland within your brain, and the pituitary produces human growth hormone, the pituitary is THE GREATEST fat burning / muscle building substance on this planet.

So there is a catch to this diet. You are being taught to grow up and smell the coffee, and understand that the human body has certain maintenance requirements, and just like that new Porsche, Corvette or Jaguar, if you don't add oil and change the oil regularly, you will damage the engine, and the more expensive the automobile and the higher performance the auto, the more expensive repairs will be.

The number of 'car freaks' or automobile collectors or aficionados or 'car nuts' I meet that are totally fat 'butt-crack' slobs amazes me. These guys will drool over a high performance Shelby Mustang or Cobra or a Lamborghini or Ferrari, but will not even address the issue of taking minimum care of a machine that is MILLION$ OF DOLLARS more valuable; their own body! Factor in the belief by some that your body is a gift from God, and should be treated like a temple, then the current epidemic of obesity and physical weakness is a serious moral defect and character flaw, if not a sin of abuse and neglect, and a severe indictment of one of the misplaced values of our culture. The ancient Spartans worshipped physical culture, and the Olympic games are one of the by products of that thinking. Obviously, the body should not be worshipped as God is worshipped, but at the very least your body should be WELL cared for. Can you imagine a NASCAR Star like Dale Earnhardt or Richard Petty putting cheap regular gasoline in his stock car? Many of our citizens put more thought and care and money into an automobile than their own bodies.

Using the automobile as a crude analogy, imagine that you purchased a brand new Cadillac or SUV, and drove it for 200,000 miles without adding or changing oil? Of course, you would void the warranty, be in the shop for serious repairs long before you actually drove 200,000 miles, and you would get very little for your trade in. Well, that is exactly what you do if you do not perform regular anaerobic exercise.

If you refuse to accept that you have a human body, and you will not learn to begin to exercise even at a minimum level, then you are doomed to continue to be fat, and you will quickly lose the health and longevity that those who do begin a sensible regimen will maintain long after you are hospitalized or dead and gone. There is no magic pill; there is only science and proven methods, and a certain maturing of your thought process. When you read or hear some expert talk about losing weight and they offer some recipe that allows you to eat bread, cookies or some other poor/bad/ worse choice, you know that that ' expert ' doesn't have a clue. Imagine that the expert is talking to you while wearing a bathing suit, and see how that visual image works for you. If the speaker is svelte and slim, and regularly eats ' garbage ', then it is a sure bet that the speaker is a genetically gifted individual that will thrive on fast food and candy bars and powdered doughnuts, and has no inkling of what a MAMMOTH struggle it is to be over- fat and lose weight.

This plan is for those readers who are ready to once and for all gain success in losing body fat, and get a handle on this ' Fat/ Health thing' You may have to process some new information and make some important decisions to actually make these changes.

To begin the muscle-building phase of this plan, you must find a gym where you can use weights. If your circumstances will not allow you to use weights, we have an alternate plan for building strength, but weights is by far the most efficient and safest method to build muscle. The combination of free weights, weight machines, and a personal trainer is by far the most successful. No Olympic or Professional athlete does it alone. They ALL use some form of Personal Trainer, or Coach, or Instructor, or Manager because IT WORKS! If the best athletes in the World use a professional Trainer, doesn't it make sense to use one? Even if you don't have the funds immediately, you may want to save your money, and hire an excellent trainer even for 1 month, usually 12 sessions, 3x per week, and use the knowledge and experience gained from even a month of training sessions to help guide your training effort for many months. You can use a personal trainer once or twice per year to help you modify your routines as you progress.

The change of environment from your home to a gym is very important, also. The right gym for you is not a meat market or a dating service, but a place where you can meet, train and socialize with like-minded people, folks who are interested and actually DOING something to improve themselves, not hanging out at a bar trying to score or make the scene. Mike always schedules his workouts with at least one training partner, and he is extremely knowledgeable and self-motivated, but he knows that the quality of the exercise and the intensity will go way up if he is inter-acting with other people. A good gym that suits your personality, budget and schedule will help make your weight-loss campaign a success.

If you cannot access a gym for your anaerobic training, we have a plan that you can use, which I will outline later in this chapter, but now let us move forward and outline the preferred method of gaining strength [and more fat-burning ability!]. A serious competitive body builder may use several very effective routines, and we will explore one of the most basic routines. A bodybuilder can divide his weight-training schedule into a 5-day per week routine, 5 days of exercise and 2 days of rest. An example might be; Monday, chest, Tuesday, back, Wednesday, legs, Thursday, shoulders, and Friday, arms. This routine allows each body part, or split, 7 days of rest, and the entire body 2 days of rest. This allows essential rest, repair, and rebuilding, which is just as important as the exercise itself.

An even simpler routine is a 3-day split, Monday, chest and back, Wednesday, legs, and Friday, arms and shoulders. Alternate aerobic exercise on the days you don't perform weight lifting, and 1 day per week rest, for a very effective 6 day a week exercise schedule that is very effective for a beginner or an athlete that is involved in another sport, such as baseball, football, martial arts, basketball, track, swimming, gymnastics, tennis, golf, wrestling, etc. I personally feel performing an abdominal routine 5-days per week is important, but Mike does extremely well working abdominals once per week, in addition to one of the workout sessions he is performing.

One of the most important aspects of the Mike Horn system is the incredible intensity he achieves in his own workouts or those of his clients. I lifted weights at an extremely amateurish level until I met Mike. On an average chest day, Mike and I would do 19 or 20 sets of 10 –20 repetitions of bench press in 30 minutes! Contrast that workout with my previous practice of performing 3 sets of bench press, and on a rare heavy day, 6 sets. Currently, I am performing 6 sets of bench press, alternating bench press sets with matching sets of Pec-deck or Cable-crossovers, for a total of 12 sets in the same 30 minutes I used to perform 3 sets. The increase in intensity has boosted my fat-burning metabolism, strength, and muscular shape and definition incredibly!

This book is not intended to give you more than a basic introduction to weight training, and we will present a beginning workout and some level of detail, but as soon as you become successful at maintaining at least 3-4 days per week of concentrated anaerobic exercise, you will evolve toward modifying your basic routine, and many, many books are written that will give you insight and ideas for improving the efficiency of your exercise routine. The important concepts for you to start living are these:

1.Get breathless! Use a safe weight, use an assistant [a spotter] if using heavy free weights, and start gradually with lightweights and increase cautiously so you do not injure yourself. Even the most advanced bodybuilders and athletes occasionally injure themselves, so a word to the wise, you do not make progress if you are so aggressive, [especially as a beginner] that you are constantly interrupting your progress with injury and forced lay-offs. Slow wins the race. When you become breathless during anaerobic exercise, you stimulate your endocrine system, especially your pituitary gland, and this is the natural source of the GREATEST FAT-BURNING / MUSCLE BUILDING substance on planet Earth, human growth hormone, [HGH] so when you make this process a part of your daily or weekly routine, you are conditioning yourself to become leaner, and stronger. This process occurs during REM sleep, [Rapid Eye Movement, the deepest state of sleep], especially if your body has adequate amounts of gamma linolenic acid, found in Mother's breast milk, borage [an herb], or oatmeal. So you can see how essential proper diet and rest are to this whole fat-burning/ muscle building process. This is one more example of how this diet works. You can purchase a copy of the ENTER THE ZONE, by Dr. Barry Sears, and POWER SLEEP, by Dr. James B. Maas and read both volumes, [which I recommend, anyway,] or just do the steps suggested in the Mike Horn system and see how well it works for you. You will save yourself a lot of time by just doing the plan presented before you, and getting leaner and stronger as you learn the science of why it works.

2.Motivate yourself to ' git 'er done ' in 30 minutes. Finding 30 minutes to exercise in a busy day is a lot easier than finding an entire hour and this program is all about intensity. Performing 100 push-ups in ONE minute is an experience in a different galaxy than doing 100 push-ups in TEN minutes. Try it, and see if you don't agree? As you condition and program yourself to exercise intensely in 30 minutes, many variables in this whole system fall in to place, and your muscles, your metabolism, and your conscious/ unconscious mind all begin to work together and develop synergy, and progress accelerates. 30 minutes 3 to 6 times per week is do-able, and you start to enjoy the endorphin rush of a vigorous exercise session, which creates greater motivation to continue and progress in your program.

When you contract your muscles over and again you 'burn' the fuel in the muscle cell. You have several sources of energy available to the cell; creatine phosphate – which lasts for a 10-15 second burst, and glycogen, which lasts for 30 second up to 2 minutes. This means that when you perform 20 bench press extensions, you use the creatine phosphate available to the cell. When the creatine phosphate supply is exhausted, the muscle fibers that use glycogen become activated, and the glycogen will last for 30 seconds to 2 minutes. The muscle will become fatigued and unable to contract any more, and you will have to rest. As you rest, your brain and muscles, and your circulatory system are coordinating to bring creatine phosphate and glycogen from other muscles and your liver, to the muscles that are performing the work. The muscle cell has used the fuel and replaced the fuel with waste products, carbon dioxide, lactic acid, and ash. They call it lactic acid for a reason, it burns! We will discuss the role of aerobic exercise in efficiently improving this process in the next chapter, but for now understand that when you lift heavy weights, you will feel a burn! This burn is not the end of the world, but actually a good sign. If you are so intimidated by this ' burn ' that you discontinue training, then realize that you are 'fat Roman', and resign yourself that you are a helpless, fat slob, and you are doomed to remain a pudgy butterball for the rest of your life. If, on the other hand, you do possess some character and backbone, and you can mature and grow and learn to understand that Life does contain some pain, and in fact that if you are brave enough to continue this program for 90 days you will discover that as your body becomes 'conditioned ', the pain will subside, and you will actually experience an endorphin release that will be pleasurable, and the psychological boost to your self-esteem will be an additional motivation to continue the program. So much for another pep talk, just understand that there is science available that explains how and why this exercise works, but your assignment is to just do the program, get results, and not delay.

Another concept that Mike uses to motivate his clients and himself is the 5-minute workout. When ever he is scheduled to exercise and it's one of those days when he feels terrible and does not want to do anything, he promises himself that he will 'just show up', and exercise for only 5 minutes. If, after 5 minutes, he still feels terrible, and wants to go home and sit on the couch and watch TV then he will go home. What usually happens is that after 5 minutes, his body and mind are warmed up and wide-awake and he WANTS to complete his workout. As Mike says, "Most people fail because they never get started." If you can use this psychological tool to amplify your motivation, you can begin learning new skills and activities that will enhance your life.

The suggested weight plan is outlined below and on the next few pages. And this is a 4x per/week schedule, which you may modify after 90 days.

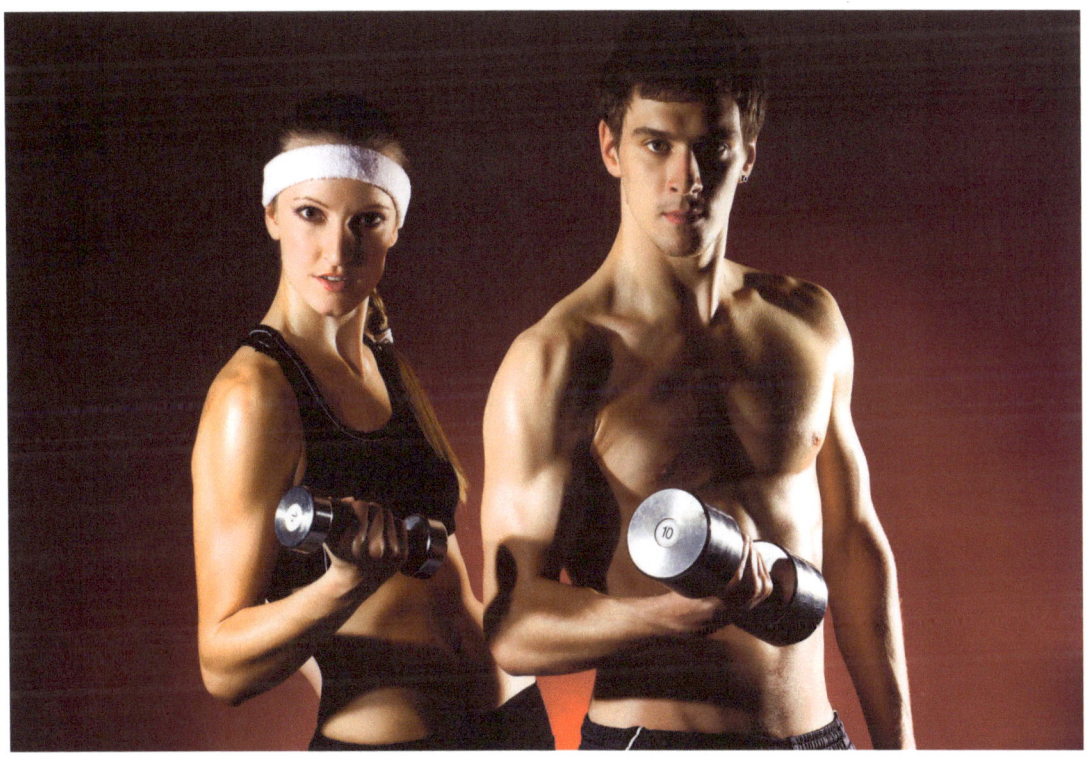

"Most people fail because they never get started."

CHAPTER 10

MIKE HORN'S
WEIGHT TRAINING PLAN FOR BEGINNERS

YOU MUST DO THIS!

This is an introduction to weight training for BEGINNERS, and if you are experienced with weight training, you may already have a plan that is suited to you. If you have a personal trainer, you are in good hands, and should follow his or her directions closely. Mike states that the single biggest mistake that a beginner will make is OVERTRAINING! If you try to do TOO MUCH, you will become discouraged, and could possibly injure yourself.

Again, if you will not begin training with weights, you are leaving out 50 % of the formula, and you will NOT be successful in achieving your goals for losing body fat! If you cannot accept this fact, you are resigned to struggle much longer to achieve noticeable progress, and one of the most motivating components of this program is the actualization of your volition, making your wishes reality, through diligence and perseverance. The good news is that if you are intelligent and open-minded, your body will quickly grow and adapt to the work you perform and losing fat and gaining muscle is a direct by-product of gaining strength. Again, you will not look like Arnold Schwarzenegger no matter how much weight you lift.

This beginning program again illustrates the wisdom and experience of Mike Horn, and is an excellent introduction for the novice weight lifter.

2 days you lift weights for 30 minutes- rest for 1 day.
2 days you lift weights for 3o minutes- rest for 2 days.
You can exercise on alternate days for 2 or 3 - 30-minute sessions of aerobic exercise
for the fat burning exercise part of your training schedule.

Monday - you will work chest-shoulder-triceps.
Tuesday - you will work legs-back-biceps.
Wednesday - rest from weight training [you may choose
to do aerobic exercise on your rest days.]
Thursday - you will work chest-shoulder-triceps.
Friday - you will work legs-back-biceps.
Saturday – rest [you may do aerobic exercise.]
Sunday - rest [you may do aerobic exercise.]

When you are lifting weights the machines are the best choice for the beginner. The Smith machine, a leg press, leg curl machine, leg extension machine, the bench that can be positioned flat, or at an inclined or declined angle, [use a 'spotter'], a preacher bench, and the triceps pull down machine, a seated rowing machine, a lat pull down machine are all basic machines and will be found in almost all good gyms. These machines are the safest pieces of equipment for the beginner, and will help you achieve your goals.

With all of these exercises, start out lifting lightweights in each exercise, and make gradual increases after evaluating your workout session. If you vomit or lose consciousness, it will probably be a good idea to lighten the weight next session. If you do not break a sweat or get out of breath, you may want to increase weight and shorten the rest periods between sets of repetitions. The idea is to become comfortable with the coordination and balance of moving the weights, and work the muscles to achieve a "pump". A pump is the muscle working so hard that it becomes engorged with blood and the muscle becomes turgid and hard. You may experience soreness, the 1st and / or 2nd day after training, and this is a good sign, this means that you are experiencing growth. Extremely sore elbows or shoulders or knees or hips may be an indication of OVERTRAINING and could actually damage your cartilage or ligaments or tendons, and such extreme soreness should be monitored closely.

Monday and Thursday Weight Lifting Routine
Chest – bench press – flat – 20 reps - 3 sets.
Bench press - inclined angle - 20 reps -3 sets.
Bench press - declined angle -20 reps -2 sets.
Shoulders-seated military press (Smith machine is ideal) 20 reps - 3 sets.
Triceps - tricep pull down - 20 reps - 2 sets.

Tuesday and Friday Weight Lifting Routine
Legs - leg press first - 20 reps - 3sets
Leg curl - [leg bicep] 20 reps - 3 sets
Leg extension – 20 reps - 2 sets.

Back - wide-grip lat pull down (palms away from you) 20 reps - 3 sets.
Close – grip lat pull down (palms toward you) 20 reps - 3 sets.
Seated rows - 20 reps - 2 sets.
Biceps - preacher curls - 20 reps - 2 sets.

Again, this beginner's exercise routine is designed to get you started in the sport, art and science of weight training. Always hire a personal trainer when you can arrange it.

Rest periods. After each set of 20 repetitions, you must rest. If you are not breathless and fatigued after each set of 20 repetitions, then you are not lifting weights heavy enough to stimulate your muscles to contract to failure and growth. You should rest 30-60 seconds after each set, no more. If you recover more quickly than 30 seconds rest, and are not breathless after the set, then you may want to increase the weight, or the number of repetitions' you improve the condition of your muscles and your circulatory and respiratory system, you will be able to perform more work in less time, and less discomfort. "NO PAIN-NO GAIN" is an easily misunderstood slogan and I would caution you to explore this phrase carefully. When training, pain is always present. In the Weeping Willow Style of Jujutsu, my Instructor Berl Parsons, 8th degree black belt, explained the Japanese philosophy to me, "the Beauty of the training separates the fear from the pain. "Fear is the enemy, and pain is your friend. Pain will go away, but fear will cause you to be stiff and paralyzed, and not relaxed, and fear can kill you." Lifting weights or cycling or running on a treadmill is not Jujutsu, but the point is valid.

You can learn to recognize pain that is desired, as the pain of your chest and lungs "burning" after running several miles at a fast pace, or the "burn" of your arms or legs after you have performed 20 repetitions of lifting a very heavy weight This is caused by a build-up of lactic acid and other waste from the combustion within the cells of the muscle, and a depletion of oxygen.

Contrast this 'safe' feeling of pain with the pain of a broken bone, when every nerve cell in your brain is screaming, "Get to the Hospital!" A pain that you sense is dreadfully and dangerously wrong should be recognized as different from the normal pain of pushing a muscle to work to failure. Any pain that is interpreted as an injury to a bone, or tendon, or ligament, or a tear of the muscle should be addressed immediately, and you will have to cease exercise, and possibly seek medical aid from a medical doctor or other medically trained and certified sports specialist. As you train, you will learn to recognize the sensations of pain as a monitor for your intensity of exercise. You may use the analogy of doing 10 push-ups- then resting for a minute, and doing 10 more push-ups, resting a minute, and so on for 10 minutes and a total of 100 push-ups. Then do 100 push-ups in I minute, and observe how differently you experience pain. The same cause for the sensations in your muscles, but a different concept of sensation between 100 push-ups in I minute or 100 push-ups in 10 minutes.

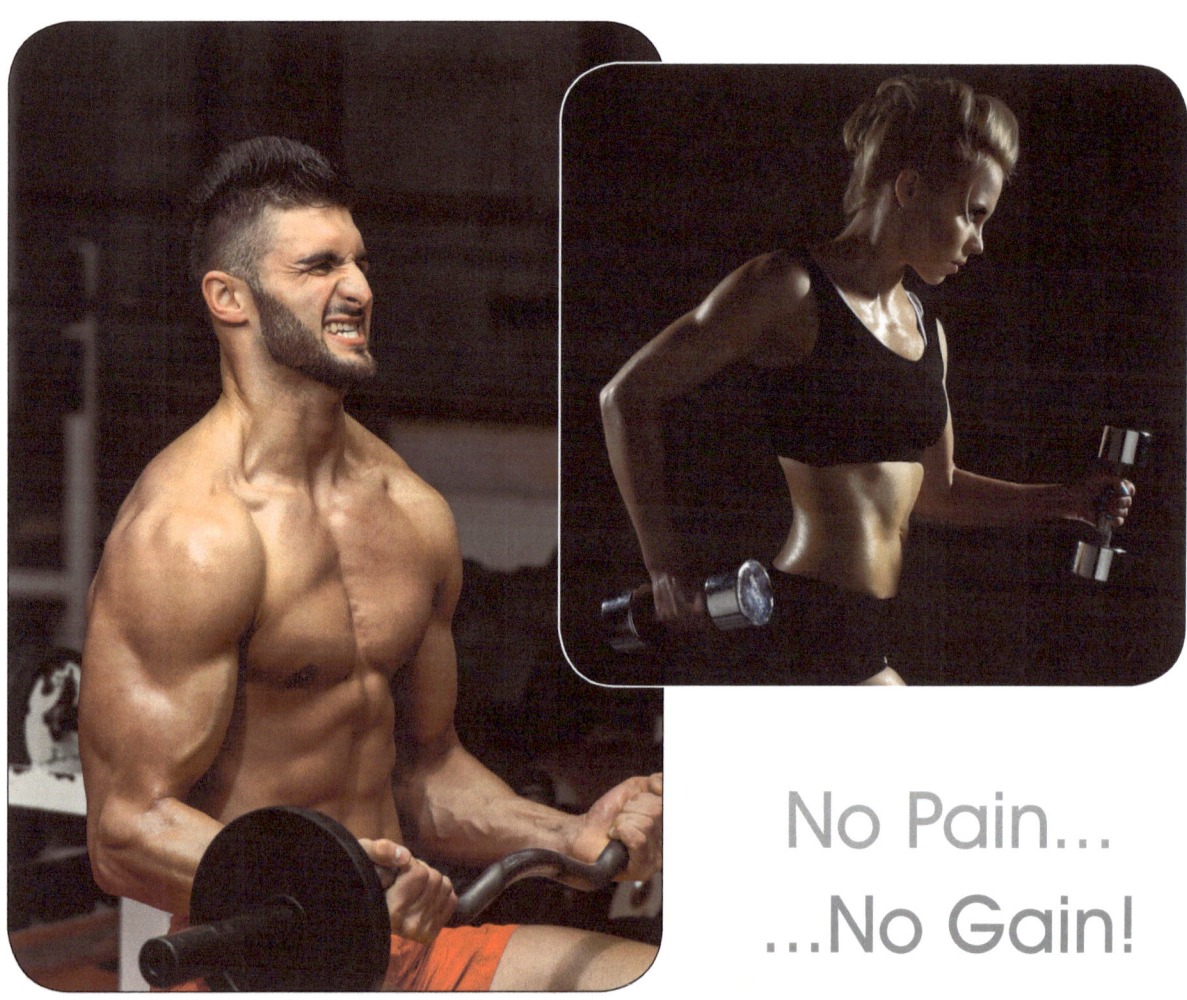

No Pain…
…No Gain!

CHAPTER 11

THE ALTERNATE ANAEROBIC EXERCISE SESSION RESISTANCE TRAINING USING YOUR BODYWEIGHT

If you cannot access a gym, then you may have to use a much simpler plan, which is outlined below:

This plan divides the body into 3 splits, upper body- abdominals- lower body. You will use calisthenics and simple exercises using your own body weight as resistance.

Upper body- sets of push-ups. Perform 10-20 –30 repetitions. Decide on your rep number by doing pushups until you are unable to do any more, then resting 2-3 minutes, and repeating for 3 or 4 sets.

You can do push-ups in several ways, hands at shoulder width, hands at the center of your chest, [diamond] push-ups on knuckles, [for Taekwondo or Karate] push-ups on the back of your wrist, [jujutsu] and all of these variations will shift the focus of the exercise to a different part of your pectoral, deltoid, and triceps muscle groups.

The U.S. Army uses an excellent plan for basic calisthenics; the soldier performs as many push-ups and crunches as he can within a 2-minute time limit. As the soldier becomes stronger and fit, the number of repetitions increases and the soldier reaches a maximum number of exercises that he performs daily, all within the same 2-minute time limit.

So you could begin by performing 5 sets of 20 push-ups, for a total of 100 push-ups performed in a total of 10 minutes. As you progress, you could condense the sets of push-ups into 4 sets of 25, then 3 sets of 34, 2 sets of 40 and 1 set of 20, 2 sets of 50, then 1 set of 60 and 1 set of 40, then 1 set of 75 and 1 set of 25, 80-20, 90-10- and finally 1 set of 100 push-ups completed in 2 minutes instead of the 10 minutes that you exercised at the beginning

Abdominal exercises can be performed in a similar fashion. The exercise that we will start with is called a crunch, not a full sit-up. Let us divide your abdominal section into 4 parts, upper-lower- left oblique-right oblique.

1. Start with 10 reps of the upper ab crunch. Hands on your head and just raise your shoulders 4-5 inches off the floor.
2. Lower ab leg raise- raise and lower your feet 48 inches and lower your heels to 2 inches from the floor. Start with 10 reps.
3. Twisting right elbow toward left knee then left elbow toward your right knee. 10 reps.
4. Touch right elbow to left knee -10 reps.
5. Touch left elbow to right knee -10 reps.
6. Raise finger tips toward the ceiling- upper abs –10 reps.
7. Circle feet to the right 5 reps - circle to the left 5 reps - total10 reps.
8. Lay on left side, knees bent up toward your chin, twist right elbow to both knees, 10 reps.
9. Lay on right side, knees bent up toward your chin, twist left elbow to both knees.

10. Lay flat on your back, reach between both bent knees as far as you can - 10 reps.

Total = 10 X 10 reps = 100 reps. Increase 5 -10 reps every 2 weeks until you are performing crunches for 15 minutes, 300 – 500 reps total.

Legs - squats 3 sets of 20 reps in each set.
Lunges - 3 sets of 20 reps in each set.
Jumps - hold the back of a chair or a rail with feet shoulder wide and use the chair as an aid and jump up and land carefully - 3 sets of 20 reps.
Increase each set by 10 – 20 reps until you are performing 300 – 500 reps in 10 – 15 minutes.

This a very basic exercise routine using only your body weight as resistance. A gym with free weights and machines and a personal trainer is much preferred, but this routine will build strength, not as fast or efficiently as using a good gym, but if you exercise 2-3 times per week, you will make strength gains.

CHAPTER **12**

AEROBIC EXERCISE - FAT BURNING
THE OTHER 50% OF THE OTHER 50%

Aerobic is a Greek word that means "with oxygen." Aerobic exercise is continuous movement at a moderate heart rate for 12 minutes minimum. (Walking, running, cycling, swimming, dancing, Tae-kwondo, Karate and Boxing.) Wrestling can all be aerobic exercise forms. After approximately 12 minutes of continuous movement, your heart rate will slowly increase from a resting rate, (40 –70 beats per minute, BPM) up to over 100 BPM, until your heart rate is beating so many beats per minute that you are approaching your anaerobic threshold, which is the heart rate where you become breathless, and stop burning oxygen, (and fat).

A very crude analogy of how the energy systems within our body actually functions is as follows:
The muscles use fuel. The muscles are composed of 3 types of fibers, each with their own specific energy supply.

1. Fast twitch fibers type A.- burns creatine phosphate for internal combustion, this energy source supply lasts 10-15 seconds- explosive quick muscular contractions.

2. Fast twitch fibers- type B.-burns Glycogen, which is a form of sugar or carbohydrate stored in the liver and muscles themselves. A supply of glycogen lasts 30 seconds – 2 minutes- this energy sustains fast contractions for longer period of time than type A fibers, but the muscles will burn ALL of the available energy supply, replacing the fuel with waste products of the internal combustion process- replacing fuel with carbon dioxide, ash, and lactic acid.

3. Slow twitch muscle fibers – slow, steady muscular contractions that can repeat for literally hours.

(Marathon runners, for example) energy source is stored body fat. As the exercises and burns all of the creatine phosphate and glycogen and as the muscles run out of fuel, the brain responds to the needs of the working muscles by using the circulatory system to channel more creatine and glycogen to the muscles that are contracting. At about 12-15 minutes of sustained movement, the average person exhausts the fast twitch muscle fiber energy supply, and the body responds to the need for more fuel and elimination of the build-up of waste products, not completely unlike a gasoline engine, The brain signals the heart to increase the power and frequency of heartbeats or contractions, which greatly increases the volume of blood available to the working muscles. The brain increases the volume and frequency of breaths, [respiration rate increases], and the body temperature increases, and slowly the stored body fat melts and is burned as fuel. Now the body is burning stored fat and oxygen, and the combination of oxygen and fuel at a MODERATE heart rate allows the muscles to repeat contractions continuously, without the build up if lactic acid or running out of fuel. Body fat is a very efficient source of fuel, and the muscles can contract and relax in a rhythmic, sustained pattern for hours, [hiking 20 miles, for example].

4. One of the by-products of this moderate heart rate, sustained effort is the production of capillaries, which are tiny blood vessels which grow within the muscle tissue and efficiently manage the exchange of fuel, oxygen and carbon dioxide, and waste products within the cells of the working muscles. As the capillaries grow in number within the body, muscular contractions become stronger and more efficient, almost like a super-charger or fuel injection system will do to the performance of an engine in an automobile. As you progress on this exercise schedule, you will be building muscle one day, and burning fat the next day, alternating every other day, for 6 days, resting on the 7th day.

5. Heart Rate: The intensity of your exercise session can be monitored and measured by counting heart beats per minute,[BPM].I will BRIEFLY review and paraphrase some of the science that has been published concerning heart rate, and I will share my own conclusions and Mike's observations concerning heart and fat-burning exercise.

Kenneth Cooper pioneered the 'aerobic' exercise movement in this country. He performed studies with American Air Force personnel and established some basic structures for an exercise schedule. He developed a point system for tracking the amount of time spent exercising weekly. He also observed that 'a conditioning effect' was produced when the subject exercised for a minimum time of 5 minutes. Cooper used a system of measuring heart rate called the 'Karvonen method'. To use this method you start with the number 220, and subtract your age. You then multiply the remainder number by 60%, or 70%, or 80%, or 90%, or whatever percentage you decide to use.

A more effective and specific formula to use to monitor your exercising heart rate is the method developed by Dr. Phillip Maffetone. Dr. Maffetone is the former President of the American Kinesiological Association and the former U.S. Olympic Ski Team physician. Start with the number 180 and subtract your age. Subtract 5 points if you are beginning an exercise program, 5 points if you have allergies or are sick, and subtract 5 points if you have had surgery in the last 2 years. An example would be that a 40-year-old man or woman would subtract 40 from 180= 140 as a target heart rate. Subtract 5 points from the target heart rate for each of the conditions described above. According to Maffetone, you would then exercise at a heart rate that would hover at or slightly below 140 beats per minute.

One of the problems you will encounter when exercising is how to measure your heart rate WHILE you are exercising. If you stop to count your pulse then you have to STOP exercising, and if you make an error while counting your pulse, (very easy to make a mistake while in the middle of a vigorous exercise session!)

Then you are not recording an ACCURATE heart rate! If you are not concerned about exact accuracy, then WHY BOTHER fooling with your heart rate? A simple solution is a good quality heart monitor. Cardiobeat manufactures an inexpensive, high-quality heart monitor, which retails for $90-$100, straps on your wrist and around your chest, and will provide an audible beep when you are exercising below OR above your target heart rate, [silent when you are exercising in you're your desired heart rate range], give you a constant visual read-out, and track the number of minutes that you do exercise within your target heart rate zone. According to Dr.Maffetone, (and Dr. Keith Penrose, Ph.D. in exercise physiology) the reason for exercising at 'OPTIMUM aerobic heart rate' is to burn fat, burn oxygen, and build capillaries at the most efficient rate possible. If you exercise ABOVE your target heart rate, you pass above the 'anaerobic threshold'. Above your 'anaerobic threshold', you no longer burn oxygen, no longer burn fat, nor do you build capillaries, but are 'anaerobic', and are burning creatine phosphate or glycogen. If you are not burning fat or building capillaries, you may want to ask yourself, "Why are you exercising?"If you are lifting weights, you will be at a very high heart rate, breathless and certainly anaerobic, and you lift weights to build the muscle, making it stronger and burn fat more efficiently. Aerobic exercise does NOT build muscle, but works the muscle to burn fat, specifically benefiting the heart muscle itself, and building a more efficient capillary network.

I recommend a heart monitor for the serious exerciser, you can easily keep track of your 30-minute aerobic sessions and aerobic exercise will not only burn fat but make a huge difference in the volume of oxygen your body will inhale and process.

Using our 40 year old man or woman as an example, we would exercise at a target heart rate of 180 —40=`140 BPM. Subtract another 5 BPM for surgery within the last 2 years, and the target heart rate would be 135 BPM. For ease, we would set the monitor to audibly beep under 125BPM, remain silent between 125 BPM and 135 BPM, and beep audibly when your heart rate rises above 135 BPM.A necessary feature of this monitor is the stop watch that records the number of minutes that you are exercising between 125 BPM and 135 BPM, or any BPM heart rate zone you decide to achieve during your exercise session. . Mike and I agree that 20 to 30 minutes of aerobic exercise 2-3 times per week is adequate. Mike does not use a heart monitor, and thinks that aerobic work at a very high heart rate for 25% -33% of the exercise session, and lowering the heart to a moderate heart rate for the remaining 75%-66% of the session will actually burn fat more effectively. When training for an upcoming competition, Mike will perform aerobic work DAILY until he reaches his desired body fat %, and at that point stop aerobic work, and maintain and even lower his body fat % by weight lifting and following the diet even more strictly. I have trained with Mike and observed his breathing and my own heart rate while lifting weights. I think Mike has fine tuned his metabolism so well that when he lifts weights, his heart rate is anaerobic, [very high] for 60 seconds during the actual repetitions of the exercise, and he is building muscle, and for the next 60 seconds [Mike's rest between sets], his heart rate drops to a more moderate heart rate, [aerobic] and he is, and burning fat during the rest period. Apparently, Mike has reached the epitome of his sport. He can actually build muscle AND burn fat during the same very intense 30-minute exercise session! You may have to build up to this level of physical conditioning by alternating aerobic exercise on one day and weight-lifting [anaerobic] on the next day, for months before you experience this successful development

I have observed that 3 weight lifting sessions per week, 30 minutes in duration, and 2 aerobic sessions, 30 minutes in duration, keep me at a strong, muscular peak at a body fat % approximately 15%.

Remember, lifting weights is pumping fluid (blood) INTO the muscle (anaerobic), and fat burning (aerobic) exercise strips fluid (sweat or perspiration) OUT of the muscle. You must do both types of exercise to safely and efficiently lose body fat; any other plan will diminish the strength and fat burning ability of the muscle and keep you fat, and make losing body fat even more difficult.

Obviously, water is extremely important for optimum health, and critical when performing intense aerobic or anaerobic exercise! Drink 6-8 pints of clean water daily. Water will promote fat loss and aid in cleaning toxins from your body.

CHAPTER 13

STRETCHING

Many books have been written about stretching, and the most comprehensive book I have read on the subject is Thomas Kurz' book, *Stretching Scientifically*.

Kurz details the science and how- to of 3 types stretching, static, dynamic, and isometric.

If increasing your range of motion for a sport is one of your goals, then Kurz' book is a must. Another excellent book teaching stretching is Barry Sear's 3rd book, *The Anti-Inflammatory Zone*, has an excellent chapter teaching some very simple and effective stretching exercises.

The stretches presented in this book will be a simple warm-up routine based on Hatha Yoga, and stretches performed immediately after performing a weight lifting exercise.

Daily warm-up:

This is daily routine that is gentle and very beneficial for health and flexibility. Many books have been written about Yoga, and this book is intended to only give enough information to get the reader started on a daily and weekly routine that will promote general health and become habit.

1. Sitting stretch- sitting upright, both legs straight gently grasp feet and hold this position, motionless, for 20 –60 seconds.

Stretches are designed to safely lengthen the muscle by manually pulling a limb or body part to an elongated position and holding it still until the MYOPHASIC REFLEX is activated, [usually 20 seconds or longer] and then the nerve sensors will allow the muscle to relax, and stretch the fibers to a new length. Therefore, hold each stretch for a minimum of 20 seconds, preferably 60 seconds.

2. Bent –leg stretch- sitting upright, bend one leg at the knee, placing the sole of the foot against the inside of the straight leg. Hold 20-60 seconds and switch legs, and then pull both feet together at your groin, pressing your knees GENTLY toward the floor. Hold 20-60 seconds.

3. Spread your legs wide, holding one foot with hands, 20-60 seconds, switch to the other foot, 20-60 seconds, then reach toward the middle between both feet for 20-60 seconds.

4. Spinal twist, sitting, bend right leg at the knee, right foot placed against the inside if the left thigh and toward the groin. The left foot is placed over the right thigh with left foot flat on the floor. Right elbow reaches behind the left knee, gently twist, and hold for 20-6- seconds. SWITCH and perform same stretch in mirror image / opposite position.

5. Cobra posture- lie on stomach hands under the chin, Slowly raise the head upward, straightening the arms, looking over toward the ceiling and toward your feet,

6. Bow posture-hold ankles in each hand, raising head and feet up toward the ceiling. Hold 20 to 60 seconds.

7. Shoulder stand- lie on back, feet raised upwards so that legs and trunk are inverted and pointing toward the ceiling. Brace elbows on floor behind your back, with palms supporting your back. Hold posture for 20-60 seconds, or longer. This posture has many benefits, maintaining blood flow and stimulating the spine and stimulating the thyroid gland [located at the base of the throat], and stimulating the circulatory system. The thyroid gland produces a hormone that helps regulate the body's metabolism.

8. Wheel posture- lie on back, gently perform an upside –down push-up. Hold for 20-6- seconds.

9. Beach ball - stand upright and hold arms in front of body as if you were holding a beach ball. Slowly twist trunk to the right, then left, gently trying to reach farther and farther, increasing your range of motion as you twist back and forth, from one side to the other.

10. Standing upright-reach down, bending down and touching the toes, gently holding the stretch, and increasing the extension by reaching first with fingers, then knuckles, then palms, trying to increase the range of motion.

11. Dynamic stretches, front. Stand with feet shoulder wide. And gently lift right toe to right hand [held upright at shoulder level] 10 times, and then switch to left side for 10 repetitions.

12. Dynamic stretches-side. Stand with feet shoulder wide, lift right foot sideways, holding right foot with toes in a horizontal position, not toes pointing upward or vertically.

This is a daily dozen that should be performed every morning, for as short a time as 5 minutes, or as long as 30 minutes, depending on how long you hold each stretch. This is a great warm-up with many benefits that will promote health and flexibility.

Mike insists that his clients stretch immediately after performing a set of lifts. After bench press, or pec deck, or cable crossovers, Mike will have his client stretch the elbow against a machine or wall or column or post, stretching the pectoral muscle that is now filled with blood. This is an ideal time to stretch this muscle. The muscle is warm, filled with blood, and very safe to stretch. The tissue is very pliant and flexible, and when you stretch a muscle that is pumped full of blood, you lengthen the fiber, and make more room for blood to fill the muscle as the blood is pumped into the muscle as the muscle works to failure. This practice helps the muscle develop a fuller shape. The design and shape of the muscle is determined by the function of the muscle, and as the muscle becomes stronger, it becomes more able to function, or contract and pull a bone or limb from one position to another.

When doing leg exercises, Mike has the client put his/her foot up in a bench or chair, and lean forward, holding the position for 20-60 seconds. Another stretch is to put your foot up on a bench or chair, bending the knee and pulling the foot toward your groin, and pressing your knee down and away from yourself. Again, hold for 20-60 seconds.

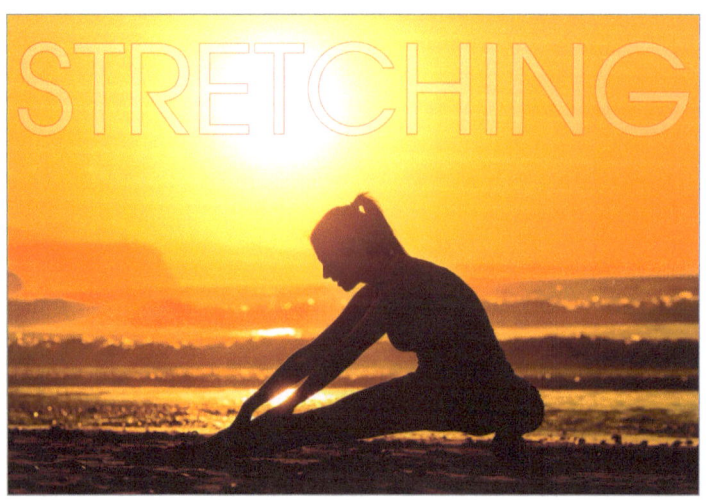

CHAPTER 14

MENU PLANNING

Planning your own menu is an essential skill you must learn to master, or else you are hostage to eating food that someone else is preparing. I think that a Man's ability to cook is a sign of his manhood. A man that cannot cook cannot control what he eats. Early man had to hunt AND cook his food to survive.

I'm not talking about cooking French pastry, or any other decadent, fatty, sugary, comfort food. I'm talking about preparing salads, vegetables, some grains, fish, chicken, beef, pork, and wild game, mushrooms, nuts and seeds, and food that has nutritional value AND flavor, as well as aroma and an attractive color and appearance. Preparing food is part of the satisfaction of the entire experience of eating. Hunting the meat, catching the fish, growing the vegetables, picking the fruit, and all the preparation, washing, peeling, scaling, cleaning, butchering, and cooking, and serving the food, as well as cleaning up afterwards are all important actions in our consciousness.

Each meal should contain a good quality protein, a high fiber carbohydrate, and enough fiber or roughage to fill your stomach. Flavor is essential, also, and you can experiment with many herbs and spices, and many new cooking products that can naturally or synthetically provide many interesting flavors that can provide much variety to your menu. Dr. Sears states that the average person eats approximately 10 different meals per week, 10 favorite dishes that we eat over and over again. Assigning proper care to the ritual of eating, saying thanks to God when sitting down to eat elevates the meal to a special place in our day, and helps us to develop our awareness of the wonder and beauty of life, and what a blessing is good food, good health, and all the things in our life for which we should be grateful.

At the back of this book is a section that you may use to journal your meals, your exercise routines, and how you FEEL and how PRODUCTIVE you were on that day. This journal can assist you in identifying the meals and routines that are best for you. You want to establish a pattern of eating, exercising, and resting that keeps you energetic and healthy, and is the most efficient system for you to lose body fat, build and repair muscle, and achieve your goals in life.

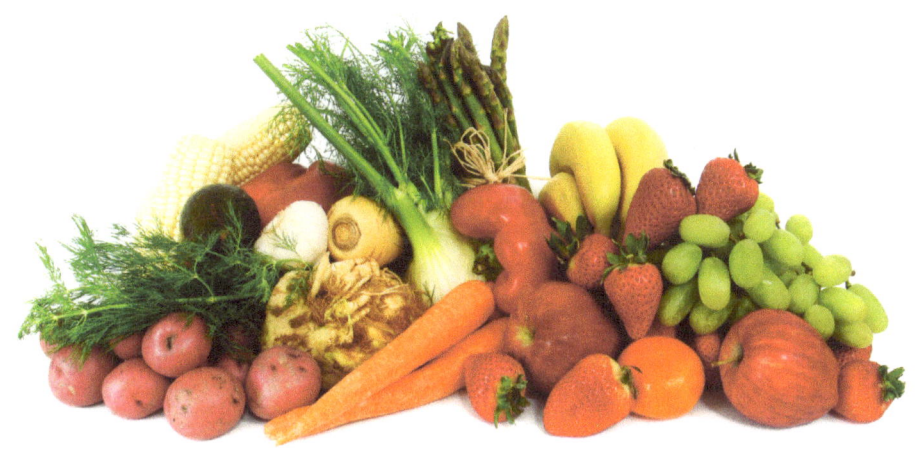

CHAPTER 15

SPIRITUAL TRAINING
ESSENTIAL FOR TOTAL HEALTH, SUCCESS, AND HARMONY

Spiritual training is an essential component of success for any endeavor. Cheerleaders are an example of an organized cultural effort to raise the spirits of the team. Cheerleaders are employed to "raise spirits." For an individual effort like losing weight, you probably will not have a cheerleading squad. You will probably not have a fiery coach to give you a pre-game or half-time "pep talk "either. Mike and I both want to encourage you to begin some type of daily spiritual exercise, meditation, Bible study, a 12 step program, a prayer closet time, or some regular practice that centers your consciousness away from ego gratification toward awareness of God, or at least helping others.

Meditation is a powerful training for your spiritual progress. Many books are written that can guide you on the right path to learn to meditate, but basically you want to retire to a quiet, secluded place, and center your thoughts on one positive thought or prayer, and repeat this thought over and over again. [This is known as a mantra] When you do this, you eliminate much stress from your daily routine, and your physical body slows down in compliance with slowing your thought process, and you can recharge your batteries and achieve some very efficient rest.

You are also programming very powerful positive thoughts to employ when; inevitably, you are confronted with the normal stresses and challenges and problems of daily living. Without a daily [for me, morning,] spiritual exercise routine, I respond to every event as a crisis, which makes me less effective as performing as the person God created me to be.

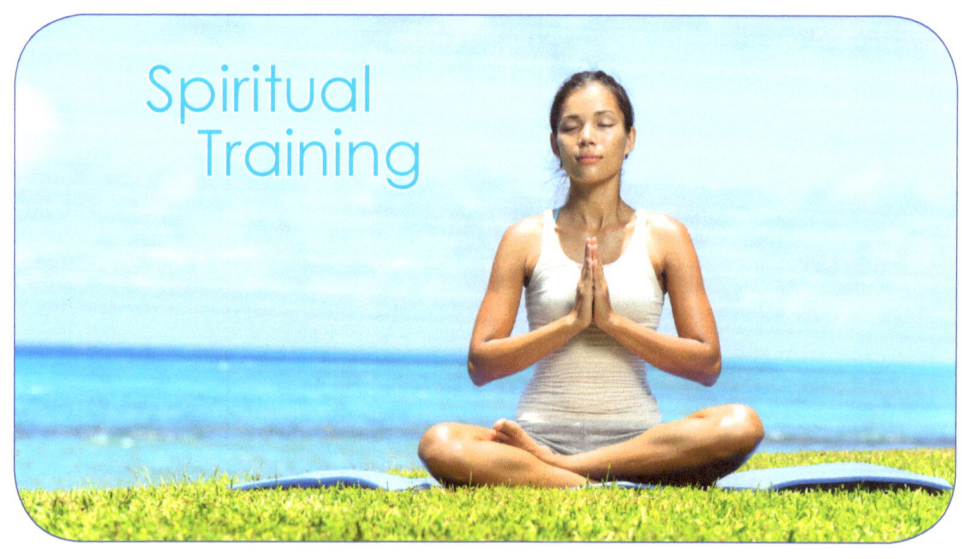

CHAPTER 16

THE JOURNAL

This section of "THE DIET "is the daily journal that you may copy and use to record and monitor; what you eat and how often, you're exercise session, and how you rested that day or evening. Included is a verse from the source of our Judeo-Christian heritage, the Bible. Even if you do not consider yourself a Christian, please read the verse, and be open-minded and logical. The purpose of the verse is to inspire you to remain firm in your resolve, not only to stick to " THE DIET ", but also use the verse as a prayer, or mantra, or a positive slogan or tape-loop to fill your head with POSITIVE THOUGHTS. If you replace negative thoughts and words and actions with positive thoughts, words, and actions, you will attract positive elements of the universe TOWARD you and you will be less likely to subconsciously repeat negative or self-defeating thoughts and words to yourself and the people around you.

An added bonus of the verse is you may 'coincidentally' observe that many 'random 'events of your day will somehow relate in interesting and relevant ways as you concentrate on the meaning of the verse. An additional benefit could be that you actually sit with a Bible study class, or some friend or acquaintance that may share knowledge of the verse, its origin and intended meaning, and many historical references to the subject, especially the different languages that the scriptures were originally recorded. The differences in Hebrew, Aramaic, Greek, Latin, Old English, and the many modern English translations are important to understand exactly what truths, principles, and philosophies our ancestors were determined to preserve and pass on to future generations. My experience of authentic Bible scholar study is that the subject is surprisingly interesting and relevant to modern day life. These verses have been recorded and preserved for millenniums, and many cultures and religions, and races have placed great value on the wisdom of Scripture. Out of Abraham came JUDISM, HINDUISM, BUDDHISM, CHRISTIANITY, and ISLAM. All are monotheistic religions, belief in one God, one creator, one intelligent, omniscient, and loving source of all that is. Many of the books in the Old Testament and the Koran have similar themes and messages, often mentioning the same historical events and prophets [Moses is one example]. The Hindu Upanishads is written in Sanskrit, which is the root language of all Indo-Arayan languages, and is closely related to Hebrew, Aramaic, Greek, Latin, and English. Buddhism was a revolt against Hinduism, similar in some ways to the relationship between Judaism and Christianity, or between Catholics and Protestants. The point of this is that the ethical basis of religion is that we learn to live in a manner that we do kindness to our neighbor, that we live in a way that is not centered on our own gain at the expense or indifference to others; in fact, we make a personal goal to help others. If you also believe that the Bible is the word of God, even better. To fill your head and heart, with thoughts of love, positive affirmations, and helping others is a strengthening exercise for your mind, spirit, and emotions, just as lifting weights and running is exercise for your physical body.

The point is that what you feed your spirit and your head is just as vitally important as what you feed your body.

Day One   DATE _____

Matthew 22: 35-36-37-38-39-40.

35. Then one of them, which was a lawyer, asked him a question,
    tempting him, and saying,
36. Master, which of the commandments is the greatest in the law?
37. "Jesus said unto him, ' Thou shalt love the Lord thy God with all heart,
    and with all thy soul, and all thy mind."
38. "This is the first and greatest commandment."
39. "And the second is like unto it, Thou shalt love thy neighbor as thyself."
40. "On these two commandments, hang all the law and the prophets."

MEALS:

1. BREAKFAST   PROTEIN _____   CARBOHYDRATE _____
   FAT _____   WATER _____

2. 2nd MEAL   PROTEIN _____   CARBOHYDRATE _____

3. 3rd MEAL _____ " _____ " _____

4. LUNCH _____

5. 5th MEAL _____

6. 6th MEAL _____

7. 7th MEAL _____

8. SUPPER _____

9. 9th MEAL _____

10. 10th MEAL _____

11. 11th MEAL _____

12. 12th MEAL _____

EXERCISE — WEIGHTS-BODY PARTS_____

SETS _____   REPS _____

EXERCISE _____   AEROBIC TYPE_____

DURATION _____   HEART RATE _____   TIME-IN ZONE _____

Day Two   DATE _____

Luke 6:31
"And ye would as men should do unto you, do ye to them also."

1. A good night's sleep
2. Prayer / meditation

MEALS:

1. BREAKFAST   PROTEIN _____   CARBOHYDRATE _____
   FAT _____   WATER _____

2. 2nd MEAL   PROTEIN _____   CARBOHYDRATE_____

3. 3rd MEAL _____ " _____   " _____

4. LUNCH _____

5. 5th MEAL _____

6. 6th MEAL _____

7. 7th MEAL _____

8. SUPPER _____

9. 9th MEAL_____

10. 10th MEAL _____

11. 11th MEAL _____

12. 12th MEAL _____

   EXERCISE — WEIGHTS-BODY PARTS _____

   SETS _____   REPS _____

   EXERCISE _____   AEROBIC TYPE_____

   DURATION _____   HEART RATE _____   TIME-IN ZONE _____

Day Three   DATE _____

James 4:2
"You do not have because you do not ask God."

1. A good night's sleep
2. Prayer / meditation

MEALS:

1. BREAKFAST   PROTEIN _____   CARBOHYDRATE _____
   FAT _____   WATER _____

2. 2nd MEAL   PROTEIN _____   CARBOHYDRATE_____

3. 3rd MEAL _____ " _____ " _____

4. LUNCH _____

5. 5th MEAL _____

6. 6th MEAL _____

7. 7th MEAL _____

8. SUPPER _____

9. 9th MEAL _____

10. 10th MEAL _____

11. 11th MEAL _____

12. 12th MEAL _____

EXERCISE — WEIGHTS-BODY PARTS_____

SETS _____   REPS _____

EXERCISE _____   AEROBIC TYPE_____

DURATION _____   HEART RATE _____   TIME-IN ZONE _____

Day Four   DATE _____

John 14:14
"If ye shall ask anything in my name, I will do it."

1. A good night's sleep
2. Prayer / meditation

MEALS:

1. BREAKFAST   PROTEIN _____ CARBOHYDRATE _____
   FAT _____ WATER _____

2. 2nd MEAL   PROTEIN _____ CARBOHYDRATE_____

3. 3rd MEAL _____ " _____ " _____

4. LUNCH _____

5. 5th MEAL _____

6. 6th MEAL _____

7. 7th MEAL _____

8. SUPPER _____

9. 9th MEAL_____

10. 10th MEAL _____

11. 11th MEAL _____

12. 12th MEAL _____

EXERCISE — WEIGHTS-BODY PARTS_____ _____

SETS _____ REPS _____

EXERCISE _____ AEROBIC TYPE_____

DURATION _____ HEART RATE _____ TIME-IN ZONE _____

Day Five DATE _____

Luke 4:8

"And Jesus answered and said unto him, ' Get thee behind me, Satan; for it is written,
Thou shalt worship the lord thy God, and him only shalt thou serve."

1. A good night's sleep
2. Prayer / meditation

MEALS:

1. BREAKFAST   PROTEIN _____   CARBOHYDRATE _____
                   FAT _____   WATER _____

2. 2nd MEAL   PROTEIN _____   CARBOHYDRATE_____

3. 3rd MEAL _____ " _____ " _____

4. LUNCH _____

5. 5th MEAL _____

6. 6th MEAL _____

7. 7th MEAL _____

8. SUPPER _____

9. 9th MEAL_____

10.   10th MEAL _____

11.   11th MEAL _____

12.   12th MEAL _____

     EXERCISE — WEIGHTS-BODY PARTS_____

     SETS _____   REPS _____

     EXERCISE _____   AEROBIC TYPE_____

     DURATION _____   HEART RATE _____   TIME-IN ZONE _____

Day Six   DATE _____

1. A good night's sleep
2. Prayer / meditation

MEALS:

1. BREAKFAST   PROTEIN _____   CARBOHYDRATE _____
              FAT _____   WATER _____

2. 2nd MEAL   PROTEIN _____   CARBOHYDRATE_____

3. 3rd MEAL _____ " _____ " _____

4. LUNCH _____

5. 5th MEAL _____

6. 6th MEAL _____

7. 7th MEAL _____

8. SUPPER _____

9. 9th MEAL_____

10.   10th MEAL _____

11.   11th MEAL _____

12.   12th MEAL _____

    EXERCISE — WEIGHTS-BODY PARTS_____

    SETS _____   REPS _____

    EXERCISE _____   AEROBIC TYPE_____

    DURATION _____   HEART RATE _____   TIME-IN ZONE _____

Day Seven   DATE _____

Hebrews 11:1
"Now faith is the substance of things hoped for,
the evidence of things not seen."

1. A good night's sleep   2. Prayer / meditation

MEALS:

1. BREAKFAST   PROTEIN _____ CARBOHYDRATE _____
   FAT _____ WATER _____

2. 2nd MEAL   PROTEIN _____ CARBOHYDRATE_____

3. 3rd MEAL _____ " _____ " _____

4. LUNCH _____

5. 5th MEAL _____

6. 6th MEAL _____

7. 7th MEAL _____

8. SUPPER _____

9. 9th MEAL _____

10. 10th MEAL _____

11. 11th MEAL _____

12. 12th MEAL _____

   EXERCISE — WEIGHTS-BODY PARTS_____

   SETS _____ REPS _____

   EXERCISE _____ AEROBIC TYPE_____

   DURATION _____ HEART RATE _____ TIME-IN ZONE _____

Day Eight   DATE _____

Proverbs 21:31

" The horse is prepared against the day of battle: but safety is of the Lord."

1. A good night's sleep   2. Prayer / meditation

MEALS:

1. BREAKFAST   PROTEIN _____ CARBOHYDRATE _____
   FAT _____ WATER _____

2. 2nd MEAL   PROTEIN _____ CARBOHYDRATE_____

3. 3rd MEAL _____ " _____ " _____

4. LUNCH _____

5. 5th MEAL _____

6. 6th MEAL _____

7. 7th MEAL _____

8. SUPPER _____

9. 9th MEAL_____

10. 10th MEAL _____

11. 11th MEAL _____

12. 12th MEAL _____

EXERCISE — WEIGHTS-BODY PARTS_____

SETS _____ REPS _____

EXERCISE _____ AEROBIC TYPE_____

DURATION _____ HEART RATE _____ TIME-IN ZONE _____

Day Nine   DATE _____

Philippians 4:6

"Do not be anxious about anything, but, in everything, by prayer,
and petition, with thanksgiving, present your request to God."

1. A good night's sleep
2. Prayer / meditation

MEALS:

1. BREAKFAST   PROTEIN _____   CARBOHYDRATE _____
   FAT _____   WATER _____

2. 2nd MEAL   PROTEIN _____   CARBOHYDRATE_____

3. 3rd MEAL _____ " _____ " _____

4. LUNCH _____

5. 5th MEAL _____

6. 6th MEAL _____

7. 7th MEAL _____

8. SUPPER _____

9. 9th MEAL_____

10. 10th MEAL _____

11. 11th MEAL _____

12. 12th MEAL _____

EXERCISE — WEIGHTS-BODY PARTS_____

SETS _____   REPS _____

EXERCISE _____   AEROBIC TYPE_____

DURATION _____   HEART RATE _____   TIME-IN ZONE _____

Day Ten DATE _____

Matthew 15: 11

"Not that which goeth into the mouth defileth a man, but that which cometh out of the mouth, that defileth a man."

1. A good night's sleep
2. Prayer / meditation

MEALS:

1. BREAKFAST   PROTEIN _____   CARBOHYDRATE _____
                     FAT _____   WATER _____

2. 2nd MEAL   PROTEIN _____   CARBOHYDRATE_____

3. 3rd MEAL _____ " _____ " _____

4. LUNCH _____

5. 5th MEAL _____

6. 6th MEAL _____

7. 7th MEAL _____

8. SUPPER _____

9. 9th MEAL_____

10. 10th MEAL _____

11. 11th MEAL _____

12. 12th MEAL _____

    EXERCISE — WEIGHTS-BODY PARTS_____

    SETS _____ REPS _____

    EXERCISE _____ AEROBIC TYPE_____

    DURATION _____ HEART RATE _____ TIME-IN ZONE _____

Day Eleven DATE _____

I Corinthians 3:16
" Know ye not that ye are the temple of God, and the spirit of God dwelleth in you?"

1. A good night's sleep
2. Prayer / meditation

MEALS:

1. BREAKFAST   PROTEIN _____   CARBOHYDRATE _____
                     FAT _____   WATER _____

2. 2nd MEAL   PROTEIN _____   CARBOHYDRATE_____

3. 3rd MEAL _____ " _____ " _____

4. LUNCH _____

5. 5th MEAL _____

6. 6th MEAL _____

7. 7th MEAL _____

8. SUPPER _____

9. 9th MEAL_____

10. 10th MEAL _____

11. 11th MEAL _____

12. 12th MEAL _____

    EXERCISE — WEIGHTS-BODY PARTS_____

    SETS _____   REPS _____

    EXERCISE _____   AEROBIC TYPE_____

    DURATION _____   HEART RATE _____   TIME-IN ZONE _____

Day Twelve   DATE _____

MEALS:

1. BREAKFAST   PROTEIN _____ CARBOHYDRATE _____
   FAT _____ WATER _____

2. 2nd MEAL   PROTEIN _____ CARBOHYDRATE_____

3. 3rd MEAL _____ " _____ " _____

4. LUNCH _____

5. 5th MEAL _____

6. 6th MEAL _____

7. 7th MEAL _____

8. SUPPER _____

9. 9th MEAL_____

10.   10th MEAL _____

11.   11th MEAL _____

12.   12th MEAL _____

EXERCISE — WEIGHTS-BODY PARTS_____

SETS _____ REPS _____

EXERCISE _____ AEROBIC TYPE_____

DURATION _____ HEART RATE _____ TIME-IN ZONE _____

Day Thirteen   DATE _____

Psalm 46:10

" Be still and know that I am God."

1. A good night's sleep
2. Prayer / meditation

MEALS:

1. BREAKFAST   PROTEIN _____   CARBOHYDRATE _____
   FAT _____   WATER _____

2. 2nd MEAL   PROTEIN _____   CARBOHYDRATE_____

3. 3rd MEAL _____ " _____ " _____

4. LUNCH _____

5. 5th MEAL _____

6. 6th MEAL _____

7. 7th MEAL _____

8. SUPPER _____

9. 9th MEAL _____

10. 10th MEAL _____

11. 11th MEAL _____

12. 12th MEAL _____

   EXERCISE — WEIGHTS-BODY PARTS_____

   SETS _____   REPS _____

   EXERCISE _____   AEROBIC TYPE_____

   DURATION _____   HEART RATE _____   TIME-IN ZONE _____

Day Fourteen   DATE _____

Galatians 5:22-23

23. " But the fruit of the spirit is love, joy, peace, longsuffering, gentleness, goodness, faith,"
24. " Meekness, temperance, against such there is no law."

1. A good night's sleep
2. Prayer / meditation

MEALS:

1. BREAKFAST   PROTEIN _____   CARBOHYDRATE _____
   FAT _____   WATER _____

2. 2nd MEAL   PROTEIN _____   CARBOHYDRATE_____

3. 3rd MEAL _____ " _____ " _____

4. LUNCH _____

5. 5th MEAL _____

6. 6th MEAL _____

7. 7th MEAL _____

8. SUPPER _____

9. 9th MEAL_____

10. 10th MEAL _____

11. 11th MEAL _____

12. 12th MEAL _____

EXERCISE — WEIGHTS-BODY PARTS_____

SETS _____   REPS _____

EXERCISE _____   AEROBIC TYPE_____

DURATION _____   HEART RATE _____   TIME-IN ZONE _____

Day Fifteen   DATE _____

Ephesians 4:31
" Let all bitterness and wrath, and anger, and clamor, and evil speaking,
be put away from you, with all malice."

1. A good night's sleep
2. Prayer / meditation

MEALS:

1. BREAKFAST   PROTEIN _____   CARBOHYDRATE _____
                FAT _____   WATER _____

2. 2nd MEAL   PROTEIN _____   CARBOHYDRATE_____

3. 3rd MEAL _____ " _____ " _____

4. LUNCH _____

5. 5th MEAL _____

6. 6th MEAL _____

7. 7th MEAL _____

8. SUPPER _____

9. 9th MEAL_____

10.   10th MEAL _____

11.   11th MEAL _____

12.   12th MEAL _____

EXERCISE — WEIGHTS-BODY PARTS_____

SETS _____   REPS _____

EXERCISE _____   AEROBIC TYPE_____

DURATION _____   HEART RATE _____   TIME-IN ZONE _____

68

Day Sixteen DATE _____

Matthew 8:7

" He that is without sin among you let him first cast a stone at her."

1. A good night's sleep
2. Prayer / meditation

MEALS:

1. BREAKFAST PROTEIN _____ CARBOHYDRATE _____
   FAT _____ WATER _____

2. 2nd MEAL PROTEIN _____ CARBOHYDRATE _____

3. 3rd MEAL _____ " _____ " _____

4. LUNCH _____

5. 5th MEAL _____

6. 6th MEAL _____

7. 7th MEAL _____

8. SUPPER _____

9. 9th MEAL_____

10. 10th MEAL _____

11. 11th MEAL _____

12. 12th MEAL _____

EXERCISE — WEIGHTS-BODY PARTS_____

SETS _____ REPS _____

EXERCISE _____ AEROBIC TYPE_____

DURATION _____ HEART RATE _____ TIME-IN ZONE _____

Day Seventeen   DATE _____

John 3:30
"He must increase, I must decrease."

1. A good night's sleep
2. Prayer / meditation

MEALS:

1. BREAKFAST   PROTEIN _____ CARBOHYDRATE _____
                FAT _____ WATER _____

2. 2nd MEAL   PROTEIN _____ CARBOHYDRATE _____

3. 3rd MEAL _____ " _____ " _____

4. LUNCH _____

5. 5th MEAL _____

6. 6th MEAL _____

7. 7th MEAL _____

8. SUPPER _____

9. 9th MEAL _____

10. 10th MEAL _____

11. 11th MEAL _____

12. 12th MEAL _____

EXERCISE — WEIGHTS-BODY PARTS_____

SETS _____ REPS _____

EXERCISE _____ AEROBIC TYPE _____

DURATION _____ HEART RATE _____ TIME-IN ZONE _____

Day Eighteen   DATE _____

Galatians 5:14
"For all the law is fulfilled in one word, even in this, love thy neighbor as thy self. "

1. A good night's sleep
2. Prayer / meditation

MEALS:

1. BREAKFAST   PROTEIN _____ CARBOHYDRATE _____
            FAT _____ WATER _____

2. 2nd MEAL   PROTEIN _____ CARBOHYDRATE_____

3. 3rd MEAL _____ " _____ " _____

4. LUNCH _____

5. 5th MEAL _____

6. 6th MEAL _____

7. 7th MEAL _____

8. SUPPER _____

9. 9th MEAL _____

10.   10th MEAL _____

11.   11th MEAL _____

12.   12th MEAL _____

   EXERCISE — WEIGHTS-BODY PARTS_____   _____

   SETS _____ REPS _____

   EXERCISE _____ AEROBIC TYPE_____

   DURATION _____ HEART RATE _____ TIME-IN ZONE _____

Day Nineteen   DATE _____

I Peter 5:6
" Humble yourself under the mighty hand of God, that he may exalt you in due time."

1. A good night's sleep
2. Prayer / meditation

MEALS:

1. BREAKFAST   PROTEIN _____ CARBOHYDRATE _____
   FAT _____ WATER _____

2. 2nd MEAL   PROTEIN _____ CARBOHYDRATE_____

3. 3rd MEAL _____ " _____ " _____

4. LUNCH _____

5. 5th MEAL _____

6. 6th MEAL _____

7. 7th MEAL _____

8. SUPPER _____

9. 9th MEAL _____

10. 10th MEAL _____

11. 11th MEAL _____

12. 12th MEAL _____

EXERCISE — WEIGHTS-BODY PARTS_____

SETS _____ REPS _____

EXERCISE _____ AEROBIC TYPE_____

DURATION _____ HEART RATE _____ TIME-IN ZONE _____

Day Twenty   DATE _____

Proverbs 15:1
" A soft answer turns away wrath; but grievous words stir up anger."

1. A good night's sleep
2. Prayer / meditation

MEALS:

1. BREAKFAST   PROTEIN _____   CARBOHYDRATE _____

               FAT _____   WATER _____

2. 2nd MEAL   PROTEIN _____   CARBOHYDRATE_____

3. 3rd MEAL _____ " _____ " _____

4. LUNCH _____

5. 5th MEAL _____

6. 6th MEAL _____

7. 7th MEAL _____

8. SUPPER _____

9. 9th MEAL _____

10.   10th MEAL _____

11.   11th MEAL _____

12.   12th MEAL _____

     EXERCISE — WEIGHTS-BODY PARTS   _____

     SETS _____   REPS _____

     EXERCISE _____   AEROBIC TYPE_____

     DURATION _____   HEART RATE _____   TIME-IN ZONE _____

Day Twenty-One   DATE _____

Proverbs 16:32
"He that is slow to anger is better than the mighty:
and he that ruleth his spirit than he that takes a city."

1. A good night's sleep
2. Prayer / meditation

MEALS:

1. BREAKFAST   PROTEIN _____ CARBOHYDRATE _____
   FAT _____ WATER _____

2. 2nd MEAL   PROTEIN _____ CARBOHYDRATE_____

3. 3rd MEAL _____ " _____ " _____

4. LUNCH _____

5. 5th MEAL _____

6. 6th MEAL _____

7. 7th MEAL _____

8. SUPPER _____

9. 9th MEAL _____

10. 10th MEAL _____

11. 11th MEAL _____

12. 12th MEAL _____

   EXERCISE — WEIGHTS-BODY PARTS_____

   SETS _____ REPS _____

   EXERCISE _____ AEROBIC TYPE_____

   DURATION _____ HEART RATE _____ TIME-IN ZONE _____

Day Twenty-Two DATE _____

Proverbs 19:11
"A man's wisdom gives him patience, it is to his glory to overlook an offense."

1. A good night's sleep
2. Prayer / meditation

MEALS:

1. BREAKFAST   PROTEIN _____   CARBOHYDRATE _____
   FAT _____   WATER _____

2. 2nd MEAL   PROTEIN _____   CARBOHYDRATE_____

3. 3rd MEAL _____ " _____ " _____

4. LUNCH _____

5. 5th MEAL _____

6. 6th MEAL _____

7. 7th MEAL _____

8. SUPPER _____

9. 9th MEAL_____

10. 10th MEAL _____

11. 11th MEAL _____

12. 12th MEAL _____   _____

EXERCISE — WEIGHTS-BODY PARTS_____

SETS _____   REPS _____

EXERCISE _____   AEROBIC TYPE_____

DURATION _____   HEART RATE _____   TIME-IN ZONE _____

Day Twenty-Three   DATE _____

Proverbs 29:11
" A fool gives full vent to his anger, but a wise man keeps himself under control."

1. A good night's sleep
2. Prayer / meditation

MEALS:

1. BREAKFAST   PROTEIN _____   CARBOHYDRATE _____
   FAT _____   WATER _____

2. 2nd MEAL   PROTEIN _____   CARBOHYDRATE _____

3. 3rd MEAL _____ " _____ " _____

4. LUNCH _____

5. 5th MEAL _____

6. 6th MEAL _____

7. 7th MEAL _____

8. SUPPER _____

9. 9th MEAL _____

10. 10th MEAL _____

11. 11th MEAL _____

12. 12th MEAL _____

EXERCISE — WEIGHTS-BODY PARTS _____

SETS _____   REPS _____

EXERCISE _____   AEROBIC TYPE _____

DURATION _____   HEART RATE _____   TIME-IN ZONE _____

Day Twenty-Four   DATE _____

Job 1:21
" And said, ' Naked came I out of my mother's womb, and naked shall I return thither: the Lord gave, and the Lord hath taken away; blessed be the name of the Lord."

1. A good night's sleep
2. Prayer / meditation

MEALS:

1. BREAKFAST   PROTEIN _____   CARBOHYDRATE _____
   FAT _____   WATER _____

2. 2nd MEAL   PROTEIN _____   CARBOHYDRATE_____

3. 3rd MEAL _____ " _____ " _____

4. LUNCH _____

5. 5th MEAL _____

6. 6th MEAL _____

7. 7th MEAL _____

8. SUPPER _____

9. 9th MEAL_____

10. 10th MEAL _____

11. 11th MEAL _____

12. 12th MEAL _____

EXERCISE — WEIGHTS-BODY PARTS_____

SETS _____ REPS _____

EXERCISE _____ AEROBIC TYPE_____

DURATION _____ HEART RATE _____ TIME-IN ZONE _____

Day Twenty-Five   DATE _____

Job 2:10
" But he said unto her, 'Thou speakest as one of the foolish women speaketh.
What shall we receive good at the hand of God, and shall we not receive evil?
In all this Job did not sin with his lips."

1. A good night's sleep
2. Prayer / meditation

MEALS:

1. BREAKFAST   PROTEIN _____ CARBOHYDRATE _____
              FAT _____ WATER _____

2. 2nd MEAL   PROTEIN _____ CARBOHYDRATE_____

3. 3rd MEAL _____ " _____ " _____

4. LUNCH _____

5. 5th MEAL _____

6. 6th MEAL _____

7. 7th MEAL _____

8. SUPPER _____

9. 9th MEAL_____

10. 10th MEAL _____

11. 11th MEAL _____

12. 12th MEAL _____

    EXERCISE — WEIGHTS-BODY PARTS_____

    SETS _____ REPS _____

    EXERCISE _____ AEROBIC TYPE_____

    DURATION _____ HEART RATE _____ TIME-IN ZONE _____

Day Twenty-Six DATE _____

Proverbs 16:18

" If it be possible, as much as lieth in you, live peaceably with all men."

1. A good night's sleep
2. Prayer / meditation

MEALS:

1. BREAKFAST PROTEIN _____ CARBOHYDRATE _____
   FAT _____ WATER _____

2. 2nd MEAL PROTEIN _____ CARBOHYDRATE_____

3. 3rd MEAL _____ " _____ " _____

4. LUNCH _____

5. 5th MEAL _____

6. 6th MEAL _____

7. 7th MEAL _____

8. SUPPER _____

9. 9th MEAL_____

10. 10th MEAL _____

11. 11th MEAL _____

12. 12th MEAL _____

EXERCISE — WEIGHTS-BODY PARTS_____

SETS _____ REPS _____

EXERCISE _____ AEROBIC TYPE_____

DURATION _____ HEART RATE _____ TIME-IN ZONE _____

Day Twenty-Seven   DATE _____

Proverbs 16:18
" Pride goeth before destruction, and a haughty spirit before a fall."

1. A good night's sleep
2. Prayer / meditation

MEALS:

1. BREAKFAST   PROTEIN _____   CARBOHYDRATE _____
   FAT _____   WATER _____

2. 2nd MEAL   PROTEIN _____   CARBOHYDRATE_____

3. 3rd MEAL _____ " _____ " _____

4. LUNCH _____

5. 5th MEAL _____

6. 6th MEAL _____

7. 7th MEAL _____

8. SUPPER _____

9. 9th MEAL_____

10. 10th MEAL _____

11. 11th MEAL _____

12. 12th MEAL _____

EXERCISE — WEIGHTS-BODY PARTS_____

SETS _____   REPS _____

EXERCISE _____   AEROBIC TYPE_____

DURATION _____   HEART RATE _____   TIME-IN ZONE _____

Day Twenty-Eight   DATE _____

Matthew 22:21

" They say unto him,'Caesar's'. Then saith he unto them, ' Render therefore unto Caesar the things which are Caesar's; and unto God the things that are God's."

1. A good night's sleep
2. Prayer / meditation

MEALS:

1. BREAKFAST   PROTEIN _____   CARBOHYDRATE _____
              FAT _____   WATER _____

2. 2nd MEAL   PROTEIN _____   CARBOHYDRATE_____

3. 3rd MEAL _____ " _____ " _____

4. LUNCH _____

5. 5th MEAL _____

6. 6th MEAL _____

7. 7th MEAL _____

8. SUPPER _____

9. 9th MEAL_____

10. 10th MEAL _____

11. 11th MEAL _____

12. 12th MEAL _____

     EXERCISE — WEIGHTS-BODY PARTS_____

     SETS _____   REPS _____

     EXERCISE _____   AEROBIC TYPE_____

     DURATION _____   HEART RATE _____   TIME-IN ZONE _____

Day Twenty-Nine   DATE _____

Matthew 7:6
"Give not that which is holy unto the dogs, neither cast ye your pearls before swine,
lest they turn again and rend thee."

1. A good night's sleep
2. Prayer / meditation

MEALS:

1. BREAKFAST   PROTEIN _____   CARBOHYDRATE _____
   FAT _____   WATER _____

2. 2nd MEAL   PROTEIN _____   CARBOHYDRATE_____

3. 3rd MEAL _____ " _____ " _____

4. LUNCH _____

5. 5th MEAL _____

6. 6th MEAL _____

7. 7th MEAL _____

8. SUPPER _____

9. 9th MEAL _____

10. 10th MEAL _____

11. 11th MEAL _____

12. 12th MEAL _____

EXERCISE — WEIGHTS-BODY PARTS_____

SETS _____   REPS _____

EXERCISE _____   AEROBIC TYPE_____

DURATION _____   HEART RATE _____   TIME-IN ZONE _____

Day Thirty   DATE _____

John 14:30

" Hereafter I will not talk much with you, for the prince of this world cometh,
and hath nothing in me."

1. A good night's sleep
2. Prayer / meditation

MEALS:

1. BREAKFAST   PROTEIN _____ CARBOHYDRATE _____
             FAT _____ WATER _____

2. 2nd MEAL   PROTEIN _____ CARBOHYDRATE_____

3. 3rd MEAL _____ " _____ " _____

4. LUNCH _____

5. 5th MEAL _____

6. 6th MEAL _____

7. 7th MEAL _____

8. SUPPER _____

9. 9th MEAL_____

10. 10th MEAL _____

11. 11th MEAL _____

12. 12th MEAL _____

EXERCISE – WEIGHTS-BODY PARTS_____

SETS _____ REPS _____

EXERCISE _____ AEROBIC TYPE_____

DURATION _____ HEART RATE _____ TIME-IN ZONE _____

Day Thirty-One   DATE _____

Matthew 14:16
"And I will pray the Father, and he shall give you another comforter,
that he may abide with you forever."

1. A good night's sleep
2. Prayer / meditation

MEALS:

1. BREAKFAST   PROTEIN _____   CARBOHYDRATE _____
   FAT _____   WATER _____

2. 2nd MEAL   PROTEIN _____   CARBOHYDRATE_____

3. 3rd MEAL _____ " _____ " _____

4. LUNCH _____

5. 5th MEAL _____

6. 6th MEAL _____

7. 7th MEAL _____

8. SUPPER _____

9. 9th MEAL _____

10. 10th MEAL _____

11. 11th MEAL _____

12. 12th MEAL _____

   EXERCISE — WEIGHTS-BODY PARTS_____

   SETS _____   REPS _____

   EXERCISE _____   AEROBIC TYPE_____

   DURATION _____   HEART RATE _____   TIME-IN ZONE _____

84

www.ingramcontent.com/pod-product-compliance
Lightning Source LLC
Chambersburg PA
CBHW040305010626
45792CB00025B/1048